Functional
Visual
Behavior in
Adults

D1609699

10/20

Functional Visual Behavior in Adults

An Occupational Therapy Guide to Evaluation and Treatment Options

2nd Edition

Edited by
Michele Gentile,
MA, OTR/L

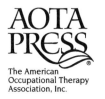

AOTA
PRESS

The American
Occupational Therapy
Association, Inc.

Vision Statement

The American Occupational Therapy Association advances occupational therapy as the pre-eminent profession in promoting the health, productivity, and quality of life of individuals and society through the therapeutic application of occupation.

Mission Statement

The American Occupational Therapy Association advances the quality, availability, use, and support of occupational therapy through standard-setting, advocacy, education, and research on behalf of its members and the public.

AOTA Staff

Frederick P. Somers, Executive Director
Christopher M. Bluhm, Chief Operating Officer
Audrey Rothstein, Director, Marketing and Communications

Chris Davis, Managing Editor, AOTA Press
Barbara Dickson, Production Editor
Carrie Mercadante, Production Editor

Robert A. Sacheli, Manager, Creative Services
Sarah E. Ely, Book Production Coordinator

Marge Wasson, Marketing Manager
Elizabeth Johnson, Marketing Specialist

The American Occupational Therapy Association, Inc.
4720 Montgomery Lane
Bethesda, MD 20814
Phone: 301-652-AOTA (2682)
TDD: 800-377-8555
Fax: 301-652-7711
www.aota.org
To order: 1-877-404-AOTA (2682)

Disclaimers

This publication is designed to provide accurate and authoritative information in regard to the subject matter covered. It is sold or distributed with the understanding that the publisher is not engaged in rendering legal, accounting, or other professional service. If legal advice or other expert assistance is required, the services of a competent professional person should be sought.
—*From the Declaration of Principles jointly adopted by the American Bar Association and a Committee of Publishers and Associations*

It is the objective of the American Occupational Therapy Association to be a forum for free expression and interchange of ideas. The opinions expressed by the contributors to this work are their own and not necessarily those of either the editor or the American Occupational Therapy Association.

ISBN: 1-56900-201-0

Library of Congress Control Number: 2005930848

Cover Design by Sarah E. Ely
Composition by WorldComp, Sterling, VA
Printed by Victor Graphics, Baltimore, MD

Contents

Tables, Figures, Exhibits, and Appendixes

Introduction

In 1989, Ann Cronin Mosey lectured at our graduating occupational therapy class at New York University (NYU) and spoke about research (she retired from NYU in 2002). Although at the time I did not fancy myself a researcher, there was one sentence that she said that planted a seed in my mind: "Research starts with a question."

In 1993, that seed began to sprout. I had been practicing for 4 years, 3 years as a generalist, and then I limited my work to pediatrics. I took many continuing education classes, but one topic that I did not see much of in course offerings was vision as it relates to pediatric function—or even vision as it relates to adult and geriatric function. My next question was, How do I learn more?

I discovered that a local optometrist, Dr. Steven Schiff, was giving small, informal presentations to occupational therapists in his basement "vision therapy" room. I attended a meeting and found out that developmental optometrists have much in common with occupational therapists in terms of their emphasis on the integration of the sensory systems. I approached Dr. Schiff and told him of my interest. I began observing vision therapy sessions, learned the evaluation tools he used, and tried the vision therapy exercises myself. I started to learn the limitations of the 20/20 visual acuity designation and the components of ocular–motor skills.

It began to occur to me that other occupational therapists might be interested in learning about vision, too. My next call was to the Publishing Department at the American Occupational Therapy Association (AOTA). It was an exciting time that turned into a blur of a whirlwind. At the same time I was writing the first edition of this book, I discovered that I was pregnant with my first son, Joshua. However, I began to wonder if perhaps I had bitten off more than I could chew. I called on the wise counsel of Fran McCarrey, then Managing Editor at AOTA, who suggested that I enlist help in writing the book. Taking the idea one step further, I thought, who better to write the chapters than experts in their field? And that being the case, why not tackle all areas of vision: developmental issues, acquired visual deficits, and low vision and vision issues associated with geriatrics?

So, I wrote my questions in the form of chapter titles and began with local occupational therapy professionals whom I knew had a great deal of knowledge in their respective topics. I contacted Renee Okoye to answer questions about neuromotor aspects of vision and Dr. Beverly Horowitz for her expertise in geriatric vision issues. Both graciously agreed to write chapters. They then referred me to other experts for additional chapters. I found some of the authors, and some of the authors found me as news about the project spread. The panel of experts began growing from my local community to across the United States, to Australia, and to a remote island in Canada. These experts included occupational therapists, optometrists, an ophthalmologist, a social worker, a cranial osteopath, and a neuropsychologist.

I cannot find the words to express how wonderful it was to work with these extraordinarily professional and generous people. Because of them, the 4 years that it took to produce what was a 551-page text, in the days of MS DOS, snail mail, and a toddler under my feet, while practicing occupational therapy full-time, simply would not have been possible.

With the success of the first edition behind us, Chris Davis, the current Managing Editor at AOTA Press, contacted me to update the text for a new, 2-volume edition (we divided the books into pediatric and adult volumes to better manage the expanded content). In this new edition are new chapters on "Driving and Visual Information Processing in Cognitively At-Risk and Older Individuals," "Optometric Assessment and Treatment of Low Vision in Children and Adults," and "Occupational Therapy and Collaborative Interventions for Adults With Low Vision."

This volume is dedicated to all the outstanding professionals who made it happen, to the readers who will indeed expand their knowledge by reading it, and to all the clients who will benefit because of it.

—Michele Gentile, MA, OTR/L
Executive Director,
*   Achievement Therapies, LLC*
*   Shoreham, NY*
Adjunct Professor, State University of
*   New York–Stony Brook*

Acknowledgments

My deepest appreciation goes to all the authors who contributed their time and expertise in this 2nd edition of *Functional Visual Behavior* (1st edition, AOTA Press, 1997). Their enthusiasm for sharing their knowledge with therapists to enhance treatment outcomes, coupled with their professionalism, made working on this project very rewarding.

A special thanks also goes to AOTA Press's Chris Davis, Carrie Mercadante, and Barbara Dickson for helping coordinate this project.

—M. G.

About the Contributors

Maureen Connor, OTR/L
Director, Outpatient Services, Central Jersey Rehabilitation Services, Inc.
Toms River, NJ

Eleanor E. Faye, MD, FACS
Ophthalmologic Consultant, The Lighthouse International
New York

Michael L. Fischer, OD, FAAO
Director, Low Vision Services, Lighthouse International
New York
Adjunct Assistant Clinical Professor, College of Optometry,
    State University of New York
Optometric Consultant, Department of Veterans Affairs Medical Center
Northport, NY

Rosamond Gianutsos, PhD, FAAO, CDRS
Neuropsychologist
Director, Cognitive and Driver Rehabilitation Services
Sunnyside, NY
Adjunct Associate Professor, College of Optometry, State University of New York

Tressa Kern, MS, OTR
Director of Occupational Therapy, Medical Coordinator, Visions Services
    for the Blind and Visually Impaired
New York

Nancy D. Miller, MSW
Executive Director, Visions Services for the Blind and Visually Impaired
Adjunct Faculty, Post Masters Certificate in Gerontology Program, Hunter College
New York

Renee Okoye, MSHS, BCP, OTR
Board-Certified Pediatric Occupational Therapist, Certified in Sensory Integration
Director, Dove Rehabilitation Services
Wantagh, NY

William V. Padula, OD, FAAO, FNOR
Past President, Neuro-Optometric Rehabilitation Association
President, Padula Institute of Vision Rehabilitation
Guilford, CT

Bruce P. Rosenthal, OD, FAAO
Chair, Scientific Advisory Committee, AMD Alliance International
Chief, Low Vision Programs, The Lighthouse International
Adjunct Professor, Department of Ophthalmology, Mt. Sinai Medical Center
Distinguished Adjunct Professor, College of Optometry, State University of New York

Steven Schiff, OD
Developmental Optometrist
Deer Park, NY

Robert E. Titcomb, OD
Developmental Optometrist, Haygood Medical Center
Virginia Beach, VA

Functional Vision

A Developmental, Dynamic, and Integrated Process

Robert E. Titcomb, OD
Renee Okoye, MSHS, BCP, OTR
(with Appendix 1.A by Steven Schiff, OD)

> The visual system is a kind of meeting ground . . . where the electrodynamic forces that culminate in adaptive behavior . . . are organized.
> —Arnold Gesell, MD (quoted in Hoopes & Hoopes, 1979)

Vision, as defined in this chapter and this volume, goes beyond the thought of two seeing eyes to an understanding of vision as the resultant outcome of a complex VISUAL SYSTEM, one that is both static and dynamic, under the control of sympathetic and parasympathetic innervations, a system involving numerous motor nerves and feedback circuits. It is indeed a powerful pathway for entering our master computer—the human brain.

In the words of Dr. Josephine Moore,

> Of all of our receptors or senses, vision is *the only one that integrates,* or enables us to make sense of all of our other sensorimotor systems. Hence, *vision is the unifying system that integrates all other systems* and enables us to learn about, interact with, and survive in our world.

These words come from Moore's anaglyph "Vision: Our Most Important Sense" (see Figure 1.1), which breathes life into Gesell's "meeting ground," where adaptive behavior is organized. This unique integrating capability is the primary reason why occupational therapists need to understand and learn more about this powerful and multifaceted system.

Of all our receptors or senses, vision is the only one that integrates, or enables us to make sense of, all of our other sensorimotor systems. Hence vision is *the unifying system that integrates all other systems* and enables us to learn about, interact with, and survive[1] in our world.

To survive, *distant receptors* are vital. Only the visual and auditory systems endow us with these senses. Of the two, vision is far superior in alerting us to pleasure, danger, or that which attracts our attention.

Movement detection is also necessary for survival. The visual system has the fastest fibers, synapses, and circuits of all of our senses and gives us advanced warning of movement around us as well as informing our CNS about our own *spatiotemporal movements, posture,* and *balance.*

Vision plays the most critical role in *attentive functions* (i.e., awake, alert, and attending to that which is most important for learning, communicating, interacting with, and adapting to our ever-changing environment).

Vision is the primary sense that we use for *understanding non-verbal communication.* (Gesture, or non-verbal "language," comprises about 70% of all communication between individuals, while only 30% is actually verbal language.)

Vision endows us with the unique ability to "pick up" *subliminal perceptions* or *clues* from our environment, all of which reinforce the anticipatory capabilities of our nervous systems and hence our survival and adaptive skills.

Last but not least, *visual–manual skills,* or eye–hand coordination, along with our amazing brains, have endowed us with the exceptional ability to continually create, invent, and discover new things. We have moved from being simple tool users with "primitive" language abilities to computer, fax, and satellite communicators, moving about in cars, planes, and "space ships." Yet, in spite of all of our advances in technology and science, we still have to depend on our basic visual–manual skills for learning about and using the "tools" that we create.

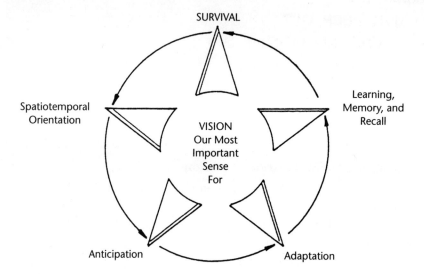

SURVIVAL
Of our two distant receptors, vision is our primary early alerting system, especially for movement detection, with the auditory system second. All other receptors are contact receptors.

SPATIOTEMPORAL ORIENTATION
Peripheral vision is critical for orientation and movement in space, together with the vestibular and proprioceptive systems of the neck and body. These senses enable us to maintain dynamic postures, balance, and complex movement patterns and to move *freely* in the environment.

ANTICIPATION or the ANTICIPATORY NERVOUS SYSTEM
Vision, being our most far-reaching sense, plays the major role in the ANS's planning and programming the complex postures and movements necessary for obtaining goals. Vision is the only sense capable of constantly updating the CNS about our ever-changing environment, thus enabling the ANS to respond appropriately to all ongoing changes.

ADAPTATION
To cope with an ever-changing environment, we must constantly adapt, and adapting depends on planning ahead and being prepared. The visual system enables us to be constantly aware and updated about the context of the environment and leads other senses in telling the CNS how best to adapt to complete a task or survive.

LEARNING, MEMORY, and RECALL
Learning is contextual, and most of our learning and memory are obtained through our visual system. Memories are best recalled when one is in the context or visual surrounding where the learning occurred. When out of context and trying to recall a memory (person, place, or thing), visual searching and "mind-pictures" usually precede recall.

---

[1]The term *survive* is used in the broadest sense and includes learning, playing, working, sleeping, interpersonal relations, and all activities of daily living.

Figure 1.1. Vision, our most important sense.
Figure by Josephine C. Moore. Copyright © 1997 American Occupational Therapy Association.

A second and extremely relevant reason why occupational therapists need to understand the visual system is that the system, because of its nature and complexity, is vulnerable to many dysfunctional skills, which can severely impact its effectiveness and efficiency as an information-processing tool.

A third and very compelling reason why occupational therapists should learn more about the visual system is that, by treatment of the visual system through the use of lenses, prisms, or other visual therapies alone or, even better, in conjunction with sensorimotor treatment modalities, they can see improvements in clients' muscle tone; posture; movement; and visual–motor, visual–spatial, visual–perceptual, and cognitive functioning.

Visual therapies are prescribed and administered by appropriate eye care professionals, generally known as *behavioral functional* or *neuro-optometrists.* A recent trend has been for optometrists to work in collaboration with occupational therapists and physical therapists bringing about increased benefit to the client, because optimizing visual behavior enhances motor function.

To that end, this chapter and the ensuing chapters will provide a framework to explore the complexities of the visual system and further this collaboration.

Vision: Beyond 20/20 Sight

In this chapter, we discuss how *vision* is much more than 20/20 *sight.* We explain the process by which people see, and we describe the anatomical structures involved in vision. We also provide the neurological foundation for understanding how vision is integrated with other sensorimotor systems and how this integration results in adaptive visual–motor behaviors.

The phrase *20/20 eyesight* refers to a person's ability to see an object clearly at 20 ft (6 m). However, visual function occurring in the reading and computer distance range (e.g., 16–20 in. [41–51 cm]), requires many dynamic skills by the two eyes, both independently and together, which involve precise and stable neuromotor control of the eye pointing and focusing muscles. We detail these skills in the section entitled "Visual Skills Operating as Subsystems."

As can be seen in Figure 1.2, the eyes are actually an extension of the brain, with the retina composed of nervous system tissue. The significance of the "in-house" nature of the eye as an extension of the brain will become apparent as the leadership role of vision in human total action system of visual–motor behaviors emerges. The term *total action system* refers to the blending of proprioceptive, vestibular, and visual processing into a dynamic system of data processing that summates a new visual and motor input; compares it with previously stored data; and then, in a millisecond, instructs one's body how to react appropriately, be it with hand, foot, leg, or the total body. This also is what is meant by vision being more than 20/20 sight and what Gesell referred to as the "meeting ground," where vision and motor become as one.

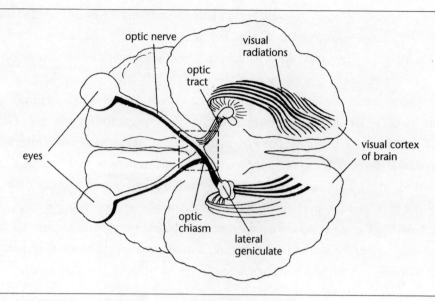

Figure 1.2. The brain, with visual pathways shown from below.
From *Your Eyes: An Owner's Manual,* by J. F. Collins, 1989, Englewood Cliffs, NJ: Prentice Hall.
Copyright © 1989 by Prentice Hall. Reprinted with permission.

A functional view of vision goes far beyond optics and begins with an understanding that vision does not function in isolation; instead, it is integrated with the nervous system for optimal visual–motor function. To that end, optimal visual functioning requires a blending of good distance optics, well-developed visual skills, and seasoned visual sensorimotor integration. In the following sections, we address how this process occurs and the components and neural mechanisms that are required to produce such an amazing feat.

The Process of Vision and Its Components in Action

Vision begins with the creation of sight, when light rays are directed into one's eyes from a light source or surface that is illuminated in some manner (see Figure 1.3). These incoming rays enter the eye through the *cornea,* where they are *refracted,* or bent; they then pass through the *aqueous humor* to the *crystalline lens,* where they are further refracted and then pass finally through the *vitreous humor* to focus on the *retina.* The portion of sight, focused in the area of the retina identified as *macula* and *paramacula,* is known as *central* or *focal,* with its locus being in the functional center of the retina known as the *fovea.* The image thus found on the retina at the fovea is optically inverted and passed to the optic nerve; fortunately, this detail is handled quite nicely and reinverted by the brain's capacity for conditioned learning. Sight formed from the area of the retina peripheral to the macula and para-central area is known as *peripheral* or *ambient* and serves to provide movement detection as well as major information to the body's sensorimotor systems.

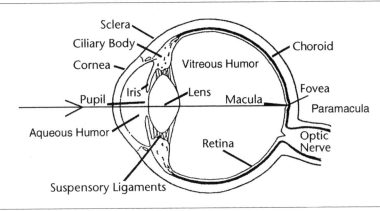

Figure 1.3. Light rays entering the eye begin the process of sight.

Once sight information leaves the eyes and enters the optic nerves (see Figure 1.3), the transformation to vision begins as it makes its way via neural visual pathways (see Figure 1.2) to the visual cortex of the brain. (For a more detailed description of the pathway components, see Appendix 1.A.)

Now that the components of a visual system have been introduced, it is important to realize that, by transferring light information from the eye via the optic nerve, we are witnessing the end-product of an enormously powerful *optical* system that exists entirely within the confines of each individual eye. In essence, we have only the output of two separate cyclopean eyes. Imagine, however, that we the recipients of this system do not see two images (i.e., double vision), just one. Such is the power and neural control of the convergence subsystem acting through the extraocular muscles. Nor are things out of focus, thanks to the accommodative system. What follows when the components work well with each other is indeed remarkable: The two emerging images from each eye are blended into one and integrated with the rest of the motor networks, producing vision.

Vision is thus defined as the end-product of the sight from each eye; transformed and united through neural processing and integration as it flows through the cortical hierarchy with a resulting meaning being ascribed to it; leading to the ultimate union of vision and motor. This definition may sound simple, but in reality it is very much akin to starting one's internal computer, with many processes being activated that ensure that the *sight* information of the two eyes actually does get translated into *meaning* in an efficient, comfortable (i.e., without strain) manner.

Vision is thus accomplished as a system, but *only* after it has been aided by numerous skills or subsystems. Interestingly, it is at this point that the visual system itself then also becomes a dominant subsystem of an even more encompassing *neural information processing system.*

We now turn to a discussion of these visual skills or subsystems, which are neuromotor in nature and extremely important.

Visual Skills Operating as Subsystems

Visual skills, which are dynamic in nature, involve the moving motor components of the eye (i.e., the extraocular muscles and the crystalline lens) as well as knowledge from prior experience that mediates their response. These skills are inherently intact at birth but are developmental in nature, with a learning curve that evolves with the developing nervous system. These motor skills are functionally affected by muscle tonus imbalances, central nervous system disorders, and fluctuations in the homeostatic balance of the autonomic nervous system, especially in the developmental years of ages 5 through 8 years.[1]

Visual skills include the following:

- *Fixation:* the coordinated aiming of the eyes while shifting rapidly from one object to another (e.g., shifting one's gaze from word to word or groups of words when reading a printed line). Cognitive decoding occurs during these rapid "pit stops."

- *Tracking/pursuits:* the eye's ability to follow a target being moved in cardinal positions (left to right, up and down, and diagonally). The ability of the eye to follow a target in a circular path, typically at near point, is called *rotation.* Note that in both rotation and tracking and pursuits, fixation should never be lost. However, it is not uncommon for an individual with a developmental delay or neuromotor challenge to exhibit a midline jump as well as regressions and a loss of fixation when attempting to track.

- *Saccade:* the ability of the eye to change fixation from point to point. Saccades are the eye movements used during reading.

- *Accommodation:* the neuromuscular act by which the innervations of the ciliary body within the eye cause this intraocular muscle to alter the shape of the eye's crystalline lens. This results in the altering of the eye's focal distance (when one shifts one's gaze from a chalkboard to a book). Particularly important is an individual's facility of focus that allows rapid shifts from far to near as well as near to far.

- *Convergence:* the turning of the eyes inward as the object of regard moves toward the observer. This skill could involve changing the convergence angle while tracking an incoming ball as well as sustaining a fixed angle of inward gaze, as in the act of reading.

- *Binocular vision:* the combining of information received through the visual pathway of each eye to make a single mental mind's-eye picture. Using one eye while shutting off the other involuntarily is called *suppression.* There are degrees of binocular vision encompassed under the term *fusion.*

---

[1]Note that, although many specific references in this chapter speak directly about children, it is important to remember that the developmental history and visual dysfunctions of youth can be of great assistance in unraveling and understanding the visual function of adults.

Developmental Aspects of Visual Skills

There is a neurological symbiosis between coordination of accommodation and convergence. For every unit of accommodation, a corresponding unit of convergence occurs. The ratio of these exact amounts is known as the *accommodation–convergence ratio,* and it differs from individual to individual. Although it is often assumed that an individual is properly coordinating the convergence and focusing of his or her eyes at a target in the appropriate manner, in reality this coordination often does not occur. For instance, if the target is at a distance of 12 in. (30 cm), then the eyes may indeed be converging at a distance inappropriate to the task, such as at 8 in. (20 cm) or 14 in. (36 cm), resulting in a doubling or near-doubling of the target. This can cause visual–spatial confusion and headaches as well as overall reduced visual efficiency affecting all the individual visual skills.

Stereopsis is binocular depth perception or an egocentric appraisal of the depth of an object within the totality of an individual's visual space. It originates from both an individual's sense of stored memory relating to object distance and separations as well as from the active input of *retinal disparity,* the visual system's egocentric device of judging retinal image separation relative to the fovea centralis. Monocular perception of depth is not a true indicator but rather an estimate made on the basis of previously stored information.

Form perception is the recognition and organization of visual sensation produced by differing patterns of lines, shapes, and contours. Especially important in developing a sense of ordered arrangement (e.g., *was* and *saw, 21* and *12, b* and *d*), form perception depends on the eyes' ability to point or converge appropriately as well as on the development of an individual's sense of laterality and directionality, which ensures consistency in replicating the appropriate left and right orientation of the shape in question.

Field of vision is a measure of an individual's ability to detect light and movement in his or her superior, inferior, right, and left fields of vision, as well as the central field, while maintaining central fixation. This static measurement of visual function represents the sum total of the optic media, retina, optic nerve, visual pathway, and visual cortex.

In functional or behavioral terms, the field of vision also includes the ability of the individual to interact with stimuli in the peripheral visual field while maintaining central fixation. An individual who bumps into things may be having difficulty with this area of visual function. Such a person may be visually uncentered, with the potential for ignorance of his or her peripheral environmental input. Visual treatment of this dysfunction by a licensed eye care professional might include, for example, use of yoked prisms to facilitate an awareness of desired space.

All of the skills discussed thus far are considered reflective of the individual's adaptive development. However, through appropriate therapy, errant relationships and misbehaviors of the mechanisms of vision can many times be brought to balance by stimulating the individual's innate visual feedback mechanisms, which facilitates self-correction. In dealing with the mechanisms of changing present visual patterns, recall the "in-house" nature of the visual system and that it is part and parcel of the brain itself. All of the visual skills listed use oculomotor feedback circuits that continually compare the brain's "view" of the input it is receiving with what previously has been stored. For example, when focusing at near distances, the brain expects clear, well-defined input; thus, it regulates and reregulates how much or how little focusing effort is required by the ciliary body producing focus. The same is true for convergence: The brain strives for a single, unified image by converging the two eyes appropriately. A simplified way of viewing this feedback process is to understand it as the capability of the brain's circuitry to effect a fine-tuning process. In approaching these problems in an individual's early years, the plasticity of the developing nervous system allows for easier correction compared with attempting to stimulate correction of an embedded pattern in later life.

Visual and sensorimotor integration involves the integration of visual skills with the body's other sensorimotor systems of proprioception; kinesthesia; tactile, auditory, and vestibular processing (as well as other information that is described later in this chapter) for the development of functional skills of orienting reactions; protective reactions; reflexive postural movements; spatiotemporal orientation; perceptual skills; academic functioning; and eye–hand, eye–foot, and eye–body coordination.

Just as the visual skills, as previously defined, provide the foundation for visual integrative function, the other sensorimotor skills can enhance the development of visual skills. Motor challenges (e.g., working on a walking rail or balance board) that are appropriate to skill level of the individual can improve visual attending as well as heighten his or her innate feedback mechanism.

Control of Visual Skills

To aid in understanding the visual skills, we have defined them also as individual subsystems, and we have provided definitions for what they should be doing, and connected them to each other. However, to effectively use these neuromotor skills, especially in the area of language assessment and decoding, it is necessary to develop *visual software programs* that will manage these skills and subsystems, thus allowing the optimum integration of vision into a total action system.

The pathways and neuroanatomy of these so-called *software programs* is detailed in the following section on the neural processing of vision with an ensuing discussion on the development of visual integrative abilities that should help provide a grounding reference for the diversity of detailed information thus far presented.

Neural Processing of Vision

Reception

The newly formed electrical signals representing a retinal image are projected through at least three major neural pathways. One large pathway provides for reception of the retinal image in the primary visual cortex, where neurons respond only to visual stimuli. This pathway arises from the "P" cells of the retina to convey information about discrete feature detection within the visual field. These neurons terminate selectively in the upper parvocellular layer of the lateral geniculate nucleus. Projections from the "P" cells segregate in the upper layers of the primary visual cortex. This pathway is now referred to as the *ventral stream* (Goodale & Millner, 1992). A second group of tiny but mighty pathways provides for integration of the retinal image with postural mechanisms and orientating reactions. This pathway arises from the "M" cells of the retina and conveys information about movement within the visual field. These neurons terminate selectively in the deeper, magnocellular layer of the lateral geniculate nucleus. Projections from the "M" cells innervate the middle temporal and inferior parietal lobules of the cortex. This pathway is now referred to as the *dorsal stream* (Goodale & Millner, 1992). A third pathway, of parallel-distributed processing fibers, provides for perception of the retinal image by ascribing meaning to it. These are the fibers that terminate in the visual association cortex (Brodmann's Area 19) and pass to the inferior temporal cortex. In addition, an accessory optical system receives input from the retina and relays visual signals to the vestibulocerebellum (Jouen, Lepecq, Gapenne, & Bertenthal, 2000). Functional vision is dependent on the dynamic interaction of these three major systems of interrelated pathways.

Once an image reaches the retina, the eyes shift from their optical mode to one of neurological transmission by synoptically transferring the light image into chemical energy. Both the rods and the cones in the retina contain chemicals that decompose on exposure to light and, in the process, excite the nerve fibers leading from the eye. The pathway of fibers that provide for reception of visual stimuli in the primary visual cortex diverges in partial decussation at the optic chiasm, which is located at the base of the brain (below and slightly in front of the hypothalamus, on about the same level as the rostral pons). Fibers arising from the temporal halves of each retina remain uncrossed. This means that half of the visual information conveyed in the optic tracts projects to cortical regions that are contralateral to the field from which the stimulus arose. Visual information received from the right nasal visual field is projected to the left visual cortex before it is distributed, and information received from the left nasal visual field is projected to the right visual cortex before it is distributed. Sometimes, a clinical manifestation of this may be observed in clients who have unilateral visual field deficits or visual neglect following a cerebrovascular accident (CVA), when often their field of vision neglects objects contralateral to the involved side. When this finding is not seen, it generally is a diagnostic sign that the CVA occurred at a level above the optic chiasm.

After the fibers from this pathway pass through the optic chiasm, they continue to the lateral geniculate body, which is a principal relay nucleus for the pathway concerned with the reception of primary vision. The fibers for this pathway terminate in a point-to-point projection on layers of the lateral geniculate body of the thalamus. The efferent fibers from the lateral geniculate body form a wide, flat band termed the *optic radiations*. Fibers from this wide band terminate in the primary visual region, the *calcarine sulcus,* of the cerebral cortex. The precise name for these fibers, the *geniculocalcarine tract,* indicates that they arise in the geniculate body and terminate in the calcarine sulcus. A precise point-to-point projection from the retina to the lateral geniculate body, and from the latter to the various aspects of the calcarine sulcus, is found. As the retinal image is received in the visual cortex along these pathways, the neural signals are rapidly projected along parallel-distributed fibers (see Figure 1.4) to visual association; somatosensory; and auditory, motor, and frontal regions of the cortex, where the impulses are compared with previous sensory memories for the eyes to garner meaning from their sense of sight.

Perception

Neurological support mechanisms for cognitive visual perception begin as the retinal image is received in the visual cortex. The neural signals are then rapidly projected along parallel-distributed fibers that often are referred to as *association connections* to visual association, somatosensory, motor and premotor cortices, auditory, and frontal regions of the cortex where the impulses are compared with previous memories.

Neurons in the primary visual cortex (Area 17) respond to visual stimuli. However, neurons located in the secondary and tertiary zones of the occipital lobe (Areas 18 and 19) are more multimodal in nature. This means that they respond to more than one mode of sensory stimulation and can be excited by signals arising from visual, auditory, or somatosensory neurons and especially tactile information. Two short association pathways projecting from the inferior or ventral primary visual cortex to Areas 18 and 19 and the inferior temporal cortex are mainly concerned with the analysis of form and color and are crucial for recognition of objects. When this pathway is interrupted, an object agnosia results, and the person is not able to recognize objects when presented visually. When such persons are subsequently allowed to handle the objects, they are able to recognize and demonstrate appropriate use of the objects they were unable to recognize visually.

The second short pathway of visual association fibers project from the superior region of Dorsal Areas 18 and 19 to somatosensory regions in the parietal cortices and is involved with visual–motor performance, spatial recognition, and the analysis of visual motion. When this pathway is interrupted, a *visuodyspraxia* (also termed *constructional apraxia*) results, and the person is not able to recognize how objects and movements are related in space. For example, he or she may be unable to recognize how holes in the shirt or pants are related to the spatial orientation of the body parts, so that the head is now thrust into the armhole of the shirt when dressing; a person who was a proficient home-

PARALLEL-DISTRIBUTED PROCESSING of the VISUAL SYSTEM

Sequence of synaptic and axonal flow in the cerebral cortex: input into 1° and 2° visual cortex, then via several parallel-distributed pathways and circuits:

1. Superior circuit ➡ superior parietal lobe and prefrontal lobe + FEF[1].
2. Inferior circuit ➡ post-temporal lobe and prefrontal lobe + FEF[1].
3. To limbic cortex, especially temporal lobe components[2] and cingulate gyrus.
4. To the kinetic system to obtain a visual–manual and/or visual–motor program.
5. To the synergic system to obtain coordinated–sequential programs for desired (goal-oriented) movements involved in activities, including visual movements.
    [1]Prefrontal lobes: anticipatory executive, including judgment, of the CNS, including frontal eye fields, for controlling visual movements in all skilled activities.

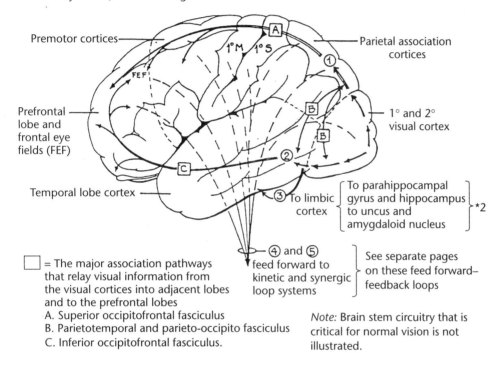

□ = The major association pathways that relay visual information from the visual cortices into adjacent lobes and to the prefrontal lobes
A. Superior occipitofrontal fasciculus
B. Parietotemporal and parieto-occipito fasciculus
C. Inferior occipitofrontal fasciculus.

④ and ⑤ feed forward to kinetic and synergic loop systems

See separate pages on these feed forward–feedback loops

Note: Brain stem circuitry that is critical for normal vision is not illustrated.

Area ① noted above is in the post part of the superior parietal lobule: *Major functions* include visuospatial orientation, sensory appreciation of the external environment, including an internal memory map of the environment and body image map plus movement detection. Area ② noted above is in the posterior temporal lobe: *Major functions* include visuo-object and color recognition, orientation of objects, and detailed serial processing of environment stimuli.

Figure 1.4. Parallel-distributed processing of the visual system.
Figure by Josephine C. Moore. Copyright © 1997 American Occupational Therapy Association.

maker before sustaining a CVA may now be unable to assemble the inner parts of a drip coffeemaker.

Association fibers of intermediate length project from the visual cortices to the frontal and temporal lobes. The fibers that project from the visual cortices to the motor and premotor regions are mainly concerned with integrating the cortical recognition aspects of incoming visual stimuli with the kinetic system. When this pathway is interrupted, an *apraxia* (sometimes termed an *ideamotor apraxia*) results, and although the ideatory phase of movement remains intact, the person is unable to visually monitor motor output, and performance is clumsy, inefficient, and marked with errors in the visually mediated sequencing of coordinated movements. For example, when dressing, the person may expend a great deal of energy turning the body and clothing about, but grasping and hand-turning components will be inefficient. When asked to change position, the person will be unable simply to shift spatial orientation; he or she will have to get up and move his or her entire body around.

Other pathways of intermediate length that project from the visual cortices to temporal areas are concerned with linking incoming visual data with language functions. When these pathways are interrupted, visually mediated forms of aphasia, dysgraphia, and dyslexia result. For example, the person may be unable to recognize or interpret the meaning of symbols, facial expressions, written language, and so forth.

Integration

Another tiny but powerful group of pathways provides for integration of the retinal image with postural mechanisms as well as functioning to integrate incoming visual stimuli with the other sensorimotor systems. These pathways comprise the dorsal stream, and together function to provide a precise vector analysis of the visual field from which to orient body movements in time and space (Jeannerod, Paulignon, & Weiss, 1998). These pathways, which receive their input from visual fibers arising from the lateral geniculate body, integrate the signal sent from the rods and cones with the brain's dynamic movement-oriented components—hence the importance of the term *functional vision,* which is reflective of the brain's ability to synthesize sight with movement. The end-product thus innervated then forms the basis for a person's total action system.

The principal relay structure responsible for integrating vision with other sensorimotor systems is the *superior colliculus,* which is located at the *tectum,* or roof of the midbrain. This major integrative center is concerned with relaying information between incoming visual stimuli and ongoing background neural activity occurring in the cortical systems; the visual, auditory, and vestibular systems; the reticular system; and the kinetic (base ganglion), synergic (cerebellum), and somatosensory (spinotectal and trigeminotectal) systems that provide input to the brainstem. Figure 1.5 illustrates these systems of integrative relay that pass between the paired superior colliculi and the functional systems with which they interact. All this occurs before the incoming visual information reaches the visual cortex.

Cortical systems linked with the superior colliculi integrate vision with cognitive processes via corticotectal fibers. Cortical processes involved with directing eye gaze and providing visual vigilance that is needed for daily living activities—such as reading, shaving, applying makeup, and so forth—are carried out through these corticotectal pathways. Cortical processes involved with thinking about or visualizing the mental manipulation of concepts and objects also stimulate eye movements through corticotectal

The Tectum or Superior Colliculus and the **Major Afferents and Efferent Tracts**
Double arrows indicate reciprocal pathways: ←———→ (Schematic)

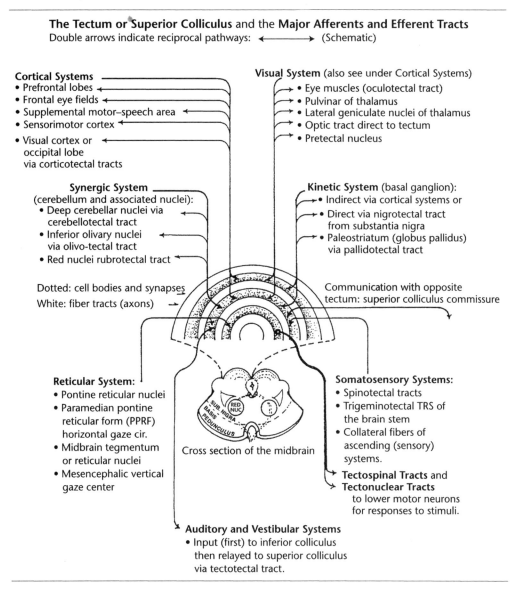

Cortical Systems ——————
• Prefrontal lobes ←——————
• Frontal eye fields ←——————
• Supplemental motor–speech area ←—
• Sensorimotor cortex ←——————

• Visual cortex or ←——————
 occipital lobe
 via corticotectal tracts

Visual System (also see under Cortical Systems)
• Eye muscles (oculotectal tract)
• Pulvinar of thalamus
• Lateral geniculate nuclei of thalamus
• Optic tract direct to tectum
• Pretectal nucleus

Synergic System ——————
(cerebellum and associated nuclei):
 • Deep cerebellar nuclei via
  cerebellotectal tract
 • Inferior olivary nuclei
  via olivo-tectal tract
 • Red nuclei rubrotectal tract

Kinetic System (basal ganglion):
• Indirect via cortical systems or
• Direct via nigrotectal tract
 from substantia nigra
• Paleostriatum (globus pallidus)
 via pallidotectal tract

Dotted: cell bodies and synapses
White: fiber tracts (axons) →

Communication with opposite
tectum: superior colliculus commissure

Reticular System:
• Pontine reticular nuclei
• Paramedian pontine
 reticular form (PPRF)
 horizontal gaze cir.
• Midbrain tegmentum
 or reticular nuclei
• Mesencephalic vertical
 gaze center

Cross section of the midbrain

Somatosensory Systems:
• Spinotectal tracts
• Trigeminotectal TRS of
 the brain stem
• Collateral fibers of
 ascending (sensory)
 systems.

Tectospinal Tracts and
Tectonuclear Tracts
 to lower motor neurons
 for responses to stimuli.

Auditory and Vestibular Systems
• Input (first) to inferior colliculus
 then relayed to superior colliculus
 via tectotectal tract.

Figure 1.5. Integrative relay between the superior colliculus and functional systems.
Figure by Josephine C. Moore. Copyright © 1997 American Occupational Therapy Association.

pathways that arise from respective functional areas of the cortex and project to superior colliculi. For example, when thinking through the correct spelling of a word containing the "ie" combination, one-to-one correspondence of the letters in proper sequential order generally is needed. This process of visualization involves eye movements even though the image is not actually seen but rather visualized. Visualization relies heavily on pathways from the memory stores of the mid-dorsolateral prefrontal and anterior inferotemporal cortex to provide the visual working memory to support the effort (Gaymard, 1998). As such, these eye movements would generally be paired with relays from the auditory, visual, and motor speech regions of the cortex. Another example would be the eye movements that accompany the task of mentally rearranging the furniture in a room.

The synergic system, with its cerebellar relays and pathways to associated nuclear centers in the brain stem, is linked with the superior colliculi and integrates eye movements with other synergistic movements of the body (e.g., coordinating inversion and adduction of the eyes with flexor synergies of the trunk and extremities). For example, neural pathways that project from the medullary, pontine, and midbrain portions of the reticular system to the superior colliculi serve primitive protective functions by bringing about a sudden turning of the eyes to the side when a flash of light or some other sudden visual stimulus occurs on that side. The substrate for this type of spatial integration is routed within a plexus of long horizontal connectivity between the cortical pyramidal cells and lateral interactions within the striate cortex (Gilbert, Das, Ito, Kapadia, & Westheimer, 2000). These pathways involving the synergic system also are responsible for fixing the eyes on important highlights in the visual field. This action can be seen as serving a protective function as well.

Input to the superior colliculi form the auditory and vestibular systems is indirectly handled by pathways that first project to the inferior colliculi before being relayed to the superior colliculi via the tectotectal tract. These relays originate from the inferior colliculi and terminate in the superior colliculi. They provide ongoing information about the external environment and integrate these data with input from the visual system. One functional example of the result of such integration is the clinical behavior termed *orienting reactions*—those rapid, combined movements that provide for eye gaze and head-turning toward the source of external stimuli. One of the principal functions of the superior colliculi is to participate in the control of orienting reactions. These orienting reactions are affected in part through the tectotectal relays through the collicular levels of the tectum.

The visual system constitutes the most substantial and highly organized projections from the cortex to the superior colliculi. These projections originate in the visual cortex and pass to the superior colliculi via the brachium. The superior colliculi receive additional input from the visual system from the pulvinar and lateral geniculate body of the thalamus and the oculomotor nuclei, along with fibers from the optic tract and the pretectal nucleus. These latter projections integrate field and movement specificity. They are involved in coding the location of an object in the visual field relative to the fovea and in eliciting saccadic eye movements that produce foveal acquisition of the object (Carpenter, 1991). The projections from the pulvinar and lateral geniculate body of the thalamus integrate images from the quadrants and hemifields of vision. They also provide relays to the visual association areas of the cortex (Areas 18 and 19), where the data are compared with previously acquired sensory memories.

The kinetic system, which includes the basal ganglion and related nuclei, is linked with the superior colliculi via tracts that project from these nuclei to the tectum. Relays from the substantia nigra and the globules pallidus provide the visual integrative center of the brain stem an efference copy of the "movement to come," thereby apprising the visual system of gross stereotypical movement patterns that are imminent and those that are under way. This early warning of movement to come is time in advance of the "smoothing" available form the synergic and cortical systems. The visual system and other cortical systems can then initiate any last-minute corrections necessary to guide the body parts so that the final motor pattern can be fluidly executed.

Afferent fibers of the somatosensory system involved with neural communication at the level of the superior colliculi mediate reflexive postural movements in response to visual and auditory stimuli. These include spinotectal and trigeminotectal tracts that convey general sensory components to the superior colliculi. Tectospinal and tectonuclear tracts project motor impulses from the deep zone of the superior colliculi to the upper levels of the cervical cord. These tracts convey small amounts of potential and do not terminate directly on alpha motor neurons; instead, they help provide for the background postural adjustments necessary to praxis, by stimulating interneurons in laminae VII and VIII of cervical cord segments in response to incoming auditory, visual, and vestibular stimuli.

One primary integrative performance component of functional vision behavior is the provision of *spatiotemporal orientation,* the ability to orient oneself in space and time that is foundational to many facets of human behavior. Social functions, such as being able to make an appointment to meet someone in a specific place at a specific time, being able to dance with a partner, and even such elementary behaviors as learning to share and take turns, require the ability to function within a spatiotemporal orientation. Vocational functions, such as not losing one's orientation when moving through the community; operating a motor vehicle; using revolving doors, escalators, or elevators; or using a map for public transportation, require the ability to function within a spatiotemporal orientation. This ability touches on academic performance in skills such as spelling (i.e., serial ordering of letters and sounds), history (i.e., ordering of events and people in time and place), scientific inquiry (i.e., ordering elements of chemical equations in spatial orientation), and geometric equations and calculations (i.e., ordering spatial relationships of figures within a sequence of operations). These abilities all depend heavily on fairly sophisticated spatiotemporal orientation. When one cannot explore and learn about one's environment because of deficits in spatiotemporal orientation, emotional well-being suffers.

Components of functional vision that allow for emergence of the sophisticated adaptive behavior that is termed *spatiotemporal orientation* are closely intermingled in terms of their neural pathways. Spatiotemporal orientation requires the ability to interdigitate three key factors: (a) the ability to maintain foveated gaze, (b) the ability to compare incoming visual data with speed and direction of head movement, and (c) the ability to compare movement of the body with incoming visual data. Integration of these three key components is referred to as the *vestibulo–oculo–cervical triad* by Moore (personal communication, August 1996; see Figures 1.6 and 1.7).

A functional skill of daily living that illustrates the work of this triad in a dynamic way is the ability to walk off an escalator that is moving down. (Note that walking onto an escalator that is moving up is for most people not nearly so tricky as walking off a

SPATIOTEMPORAL ORIENTATION

- Orientation in space and time is the foundation of all human behavior. Without orientation we cannot become bipedal, move, explore, and learn about our environment. In reality, we cannot survive unless cared for.
- Abnormal function in any one component of the vestibulo–oculo–cervical triad interferes with normal function in the other components, resulting in insecurities, postural and balance impairments, and changes in muscle tone, thus compromising one's ability to explore, manipulate, and learn from interacting with the environment.
- Of the three components of the vestibulo–oculo–cervical triad, which one is most important? They are all of equal importance, as no one component can function normally without the others. For example,
  - The vestibulocerebellum (aka archicerebellum) is vitally necessary for keeping the eyes foveated on a target during all head and body movements. This system also is responsible for gravity detection, balance or posture, and muscle tone during all activities of daily living.
  - The visual component (ocular system), especially peripheral or ambient vision, is vital for orientation in space, movement detection, and a global awareness of space and time. The foveal (macular) vision is essential for learning details (e.g., reading, driving, writing) as well as saccadic and smooth-pursuit movements used in all learning and activities of daily living.
  - The rostral neck (cervical) receptors orient the head in space along with all special senses, including the ocular and vestibular systems. The rostral cervical levels of the neck prove to be the vital link between the rest of the body and the head, enabling the entire body/head to function together as an integrated whole.

- -

VESTIBULO–OCULO–CERVICAL TRIAD

- VOR = Maintains a foveated gaze on a target during all head movements, especially during fast, brief head movements. This is a compensatory mechanism (reflex) that moves the eyes equally and opposite to the head movements, thus keeping the eyes foveated (focused) on a target.
- OVR = Feedback circuit of VOR (or eyes to vestibular nucleus). Relays data informing vestibular nucleus if eyes are on target (a match) or off-target (mismatch) and need correcting.
- COR = A backup system for VOR (may account for 25% of VOR function), especially utilized for slow, sustained movements of the neck/head. Same functions as VOR, plus links head and body together as a unified whole.
- OCR = Voluntary or involuntary (reflexive) eye movements as in supra- or infraversion or levo- or dextroversion. Increases muscle tone in muscles "looked at," which in turn extends, flexes, or rotates the neck in the gaze direction and reciprocally reduces tone in the opposite group of muscles, thus reinforcing movement in direction of gaze.
- VCR = Functions with above reflexes for equilibrium, antigravity muscle tone, and informing the rostral cervical area about the moment-to-moment (milliseconds) state of the vestibulocerebellum and ocular system.
- CVR = Feedback to vestibulocerebellum for correcting or reinforcing neck movements in relation to head and body balance/posture, gravity, and muscle tone of all movements.
- VSR = Functions with all above for body parts in relation to balance, gravity, movement, and orientation of body in space. Involved in tonic and dynamic responses, especially of limbs.
- SVR = Feedback to vestibulocerebellum to correct or enhance body posture and movements, especially with the limbs.

Figure 1.6. Notes on spatiotemporal orientation and the vestibulo–oculo–cervical triad. Figure by Josephine C. Moore. Copyright © 1997 American Occupational Therapy Association.

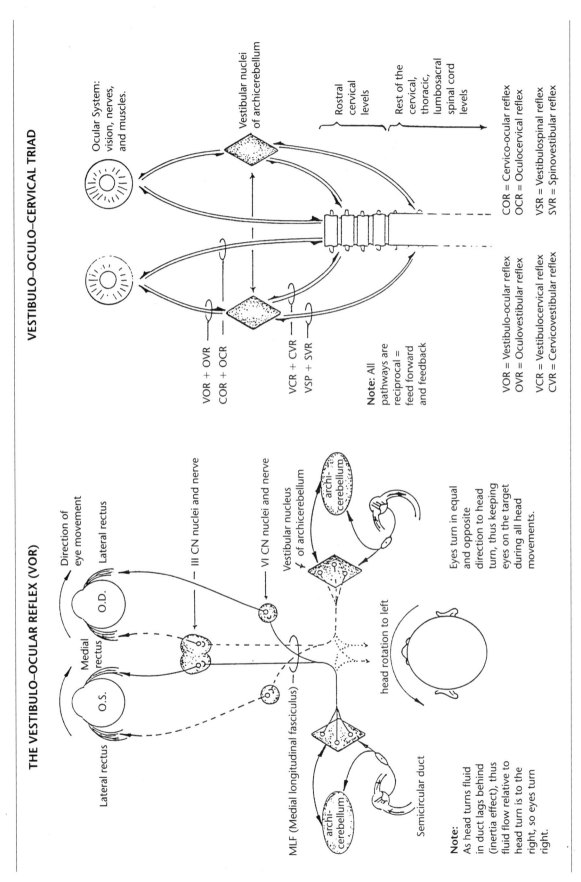

Figure 1.7. Schematic diagram of spatiotemporal orientation, the oculo–vestibular reflex, and the vestibulo–oculo–cervical triad.
Figure by Josephine C. Moore. Copyright © 1997 American Occupational Therapy Association.

downward-moving stairway.) Consider (a) the need to maintain foveated gaze on the upcoming floor and the gap between moving and nonmoving supporting surfaces that become the visual target. Now consider (b) the ability to compare the efference copy of movement of the visual field arising from the foveated gaze with the efference copy of speed and direction of movement of the head in space arising from incoming vestibular data. Next, hold that thought while (c) the visual and vestibular efference copies of movement are compared with incoming kinetic data arising from the proprioceptors in the neck that apprise the individual that the body is involved in steady-state postural adjustments and is working on standing still. Temporospatial orientation provides for resolution of movement equations in time and space, among other things, and enables a person to time the integration of body movement with the location of sensory events in the environment.

The *vestibular ocular reflex* is the neural mechanism responsible for (a) the ability to maintain foveated gaze. Relays between the vestibular nuclei and the nuclei of the extraocular muscles project through and around the medial longitudinal fasciculus (MLF) to produce compensatory eye movements in response to head movements. These eye movements help to stabilize the visual image on the retina. Feedback from the oculomotor nuclear complex is accomplished via reciprocal interneural pathways. These pathways link the functions of the vestibular nuclei apprised of the movement occurring in the eye muscles. The portion of the loop that provides feedback directly to the vestibular nuclei from the oculomotor complex is termed the *oculovestibular reflex*. Integration of data from both of these circuits facilitates (b) one's ability to compare incoming visual data with speed and direction of head movement.

The neural pathways responsible for (c) comparing movement of the body with incoming visual data consist of relays among the interstitial nucleus of Cajal, the oculomotor nuclear complex, and the spinal cord. These circuits provide both feed-forward and feedback mechanisms and are termed the *oculocervical reflex* and the *cervico–ocular reflex*. Efferent fibers from this functional system of relays descend to the spinal cord as the interstiospinal components of the MLF and provide synergistic changes in muscle tone to complement movement in the direction of eye gaze.

Reflexive pathways link the superior colliculus and the spinal cord via the interstiospinal component of the MLF, reticulospinal reflex, vestibulocervical reflex (VCR), and vestibulospinal reflex (VSR). The VCR and VSR serve as the final link in the vestibulo–oculo–cervical triad by interfacing postural support mechanisms with visual and vestibular efferences. Their interaction complements the work of the cervico–ocular reflex and oculocervical reflex by adjusting postural tone to support the movement to come. The action of the VCR and VSR is modified by their feedback loops, which arise from upper cervical segments of the spinal cord and project to the superior colliculus, cerebellum, and vestibular nuclear center via spinotectal, spinocerebellar, spinovestibular, and spinoreticular fibers.

HOW VISUAL CLUES DIRECT MOTOR MOVEMENTS

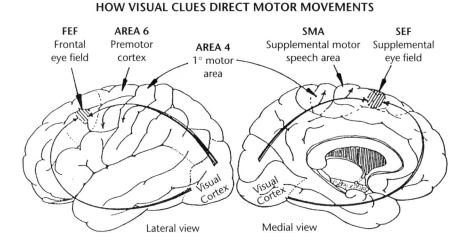

1. Direct pathways from visual cortices to areas noted above.

2. Concurrently (via dentatothalammocortical circuits) input from the neocerebellum reaches Areas **6** and **4** for coordinating all synergic movements = direction, extent, force, timing, and (muscle) tone of intended movements.

3. **FEF** and **SEF** send fibers directly and indirectly to saccadic generator centers of brain stem, hence to CN. Nuclei of III, IV, and VI to move eyes to guide movements.

4. Final commands for movements from Areas **6** and **4** descend via corticospinal and corticonuclear TRS to LMNs involved in performing skilled sequential movements.

MOVEMENT PROGRAM GENERATOR CENTERS ENGAGED IN MENTAL PLANNING OF A MOVEMENT SEQUENCE

SEF (Supplementary eye field) is believed to be the *program generator center for saccadic eye movements* accompanying all preplanned or anticipatory eye movements. This center is active prior to any actual movements of the eyes. **SEF** has reciprocal connections and functions with the **FEF**, **PEF** (posterior eye field in rostral Area 39 of the angular gyrus and intraparietal sulcus), and the **DLPFC** (dorsolateral prefrontal cortex), all centers involved in cortical control of saccadic eye movements, etc. Hence, **SEF** is active even during mental imagery and mental planning of a movement sequence prior to the actual movement taking place.

SMA (Supplementary motor–speech area) is believed to be the *program generator center for anticipatory or preplanned* (i.e., mentally thinking through a movement sequence) *"motor"* behaviors.

Area **4** (1° motor) and Area **6** (premotor cortex) are active during the actual performance, having been signaled to act by the program generator centers **SEF** and **SMA**.

Persons with bradykinesia, hypokinesia, or akinesia, as seen in Parkinson's disease and parkinsonism, demonstrate the phenomenon of "can't get started" syndrome due to loss of dopaminergic input to **SMA** and other cortical/subcortical areas. However, a patient can use vision as a "starter" if a definite area (hallway, room, walk) is clearly marked off with high-contrast guidance lines on the floor.

Figure 1.8. How visual clues direct motor movements.
Figure by Josephine C. Moore. Copyright © 1997 American Occupational Therapy Association.

Visual guidance of motor activities provides the final link in the reverberating neural circuitry that constitutes functional vision. Visual guidance allows a person to respond to his or her perceptions of the retinal image (see Figure 1.8). Cortical control of eye movements is accomplished through reciprocal pathways among three cortical centers: (a) the frontal eye fields; (b) area fields (Area 6, medially located), which are responsible for purposeful, anticipatory, saccadic eye movements to targets of behavioral importance; and (c) the posterior eye fields (Area 39), which are responsible for smoothing out eye movements. Disturbance of these pathways is implicated in ideational apraxia, whereas disturbances of motor planning result when circuits linking visual, premotor, and motor speech areas are interrupted (see Figure 1.9).

As can be seen, functional vision encompasses a vast network of related pathways, integrated reflexes, and interneuronal relays whose influence extends throughout the neuroaxis. It is totally dependent on the neuronal interactions of circuits that allow for reception of retinal image; integration of that image with subcortical mechanisms of partial control; balance anticipatory sensorimotor relays; perception of the retinal image through parallel-distributed processing at the various cortical levels or centers; and, finally, the ability to use the cortically controlled direction of eye gaze to plan a response to the retinal image, or vice versa (i.e., the eyes can move first to find a specific retinal image).

Furthermore, this complex system also leads to partial support for praxis, eye–hand teaming, and orientation, with all of the above combining to create a *total action system* that defines the ultimate union of vision and motor. As readers can well imagine, disruption due to trauma, developmental delay, poor visual skills relating to accommodative and vergence dysfunction, or congenital abnormalities along any of these pathways brings with it the potential to disrupt some aspects of functional visual behavior with its resulting effects on the aforementioned total action system.

In the following sections, we explore the development of the visual system and difficulties it faces in attempting to become one with the motor system.

Development of Visual Integrative Abilities

It is clear that one does not spring forth with a fully developed, homeostatically balanced visual system; instead, one must move slowly and sometimes laboriously through both the development and integrative processes of the feedback mechanisms of vision, proprioception, balance, touch, and audition. Pause for a moment to reflect on the systems and development involved for a major league baseball player to make a seemingly impossible acrobatic catch. Now think back to a preschooler's first attempt to catch a gently tossed ball. How did each get from A to Z? Think also of the confusion of a 6-year-old ballerina as she struggled to keep from being lost in space. Contrast this individual with the extraordinary grace shown by the same person just a few years later. Vision and integration of motor skills are indeed *emergent*.

In defining this integration process, Gesell, Ilg, and Ames (1946) stated,

> For the child, the space world is not a fixed and static absolute. It is a plastic domain, which he manipulates in terms of his nascent powers. He was born with a pair of eyes, but not with a visual world. He must build that world himself through a series of positive acts.

CIRCUITRY INVOLVED IN MENTAL PLANNING OF AN ACTIVITY

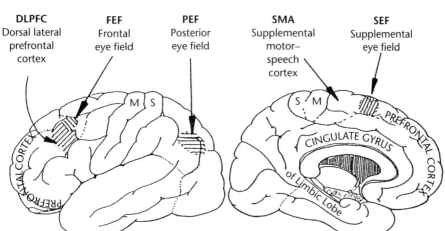

DLPFC
Dorsal lateral prefrontal cortex

FEF
Frontal eye field

PEF
Posterior eye field

SMA
Supplemental motor– speech cortex

SEF
Supplemental eye field

1. From all neocortical areas and limbic cortex and especially FEF, DLPFC, PEF, and SEF (program generator center for saccadic eye movements) and SMA (program generator center for face/body movements).

2. Via corticostriatal TRS to caudate nucleus, putamen, and ventral striatum and substantia nigra (all nuclei of basal ganglia).

3. Nigrostriatal feedback pathway (dopaminergic system).

4. From basal ganglia nuclei (see #2) via thalamus to cortical areas SMA, and concurrently via thalamic nuclei (centromedian, ventral lateral, and ventral posterior nuclei) to sensorimotor cortices, the prefrontal cortex, and the cingulate gyrus of the limbic lobe via substantia nigra, dorsal medial, and ventral medial thalamic nuclei.

5. Above represents circuitry involved in "setting up" a preplanned or anticipated sequence of skilled activities.

CIRCUITRY INVOLVED IN VOLUNTARY CONTROL OF GAZE AND INITIATION OF EYE MOVEMENTS

1. From all cortical areas and especially SEF, FEF, DLPFC, and PEF (see illustration this page).
2. Via corticostriatal tracts to caudate nucleus putamen, ventral striatum, and relay to paleostriatum.
3. To substantia nigra (of midbrain) with parallel distribution to striatum (feedback), to superior colliculus (tectum) of midbrain, and to saccadic generator CTRs.
4. Parallel distribution from tectum (superior colliculus) to
   - Cranial nerve nuclei of III, IV, and VI.
   - PPRF (paramedian pontine reticular formation) for horizontal gaze and saccadic movements.
   - RIMLF (rostral interstitual nucleus of medial longitudinal fasciculus) for vertical gaze and saccadic movements.
   - Hence to cranial nerve nuclei III, IV, and VI and to their respective eye muscles controlling horizontal and vertical eye movements.
   - Tectoreticular input to reticular formation of the medulla. Hence reticulospinal tracts to LMNs of the body.
   - Tectonuclear and tectospinal TRS to LMNs of face/body for coordinating eye movements with facial (head) and body movements.

Note: The circuits of the synergic system (cerebellum, etc.) are not included but are engaged in all facial/body actions including mental planning, etc.

Figure 1.9. Circuitry involved in the mental planning of an activity and in voluntary control of gaze and initiation of eye movements.
Figure by Josephine C. Moore. Copyright © 1997 American Occupational Therapy Association.

Thus, the purpose of a child's developmental vision years is to establish the foundation of sensory information and experience needed to direct movement (e.g., the "positive acts" referred to by Gesell et al., 1946). Each time a young child makes a foray into space, the visual system is directing the exploration. The proprioceptive, kinesthetic, tactual, vestibular, auditory, and visual sensory experiences thus garnered through the movement itself and through interaction with objects in the environment are returned to the visual system, where they are integrated and stored. The action years, between ages 1 and 6, are particularly responsible for the developmental integration of these systems. During this time, the organism is driven to explore and experiment with its motor systems, resulting in the formation of the ability to interact with stimuli within arm's length, as well as garnering and understanding of how to project and localize objects outside arm's length. Therein lies the definition of the term *visual space world*.

John Streff (1971) explained the creation of this space world as follows:

> Every time the visual system receives a stimulus, it analyzes and matches it against the memory banks of cumulative experience of the whole body/mind system. Accordingly, the way it integrates ("sees") that stimulus or image is conditioned by the previous experience of the whole organism. At the same time the new stimulus is added to and synthesized with the old experience, becoming a part of the analyzing, matching mechanism that is applied to the next stimulus.

Visual skills (as described above) as well as visual integrative abilities are inherent to the system of the developing child. The process of visual ability development begins as soon as a newborn opens his or her eyes. However, even though the intact child comes with muscles, neural connections, and integrative pathways, the degree to which these structures are *efficient* and *integrated* with each other, as well as their integration with the other sensory systems, becomes a developmental question. Some children develop normally and enjoy well-coordinated eye–hand–body skills; some become good athletes, while other individuals, either on their own or through various therapy modalities, develop and integrate their skills to an even higher level, with the ability to perform extraordinary feats, such as the type of skills and abilities demonstrated by a Top Gun pilot.

Some individuals, though, will have difficulty developing their visual skills and integrative abilities in an efficient manner. This is especially true for children with developmental delays and nervous system disorders that restrict their development of orderly movement patterns. As explained earlier, as a consequence of their compromised or delayed nervous systems they might have a reduced opportunity for accurate feedback opportunities on which to build a foundation for optimal functional sensorimotor integration. Children who experience such delays and compromises also are at great risk for dysfunction within their visual systems as well.

Although in one sense the visual system could exist in isolation from the potential of the other sensorimotor systems, an individual's visual abilities would suffer without the benefit of the input of the other sensorimotor systems. Visual abilities that develop in isolation from the other sensorimotor systems would not develop as efficiently or completely as would a normally functioning system. Conversely, in an individual with a normally functioning sensorimotor system, any visually directed act carried out in the presence of bodily movement or involving eye–hand–body responses to expected or unexpected external stimuli would then be representative of the integration occurring in the total action system.

Although this chapter does not specifically address treatment, it is important that remediation of the sensorimotor system be conducted in concert with an individual's visual skills so that optimal integration can be achieved. The visual skills of tracking, saccades, pursuits, convergence, divergence, and accommodative flexibility are notably enhanced when the variables of proprioception and vestibular input (e.g., walking rail, balance board) are added to the equation.

Visual Dysfunctions

Now that we have an insight into the components that determine the process of vision, we can begin a discussion of what can go amiss with the visual system. This section is intended as an overview of, or framework for, understanding the nature of various visual dysfunctions. Dysfunctions are categorized as *pathological, refractive,* and *physiological.* Breakdowns in the neural processes of reception, perception, and integration also can and do occur.

Pathological Dysfunction

Pathological dysfunction refers to problems with ocular health. A description of the ocular structures and associated pathology are included in Appendixes 1.A and 1.B.

Refractive Dysfunction

Refractive dysfunction includes problems with visual acuity, or optical errors. A description of refractive conditions known as *refractive errors* follows.

To begin, light rays enter the eye, pass through several transparent ocular structures, and undergo a process of bending known as *refraction.* Refraction makes it possible for light from a large area to be focused on a very small area (the retina), where the photoreceptors (rods and cones) are found.

The cornea and crystalline lens are, as previously mentioned, the primary ocular structures responsible for refraction. The cornea is very powerful, but because the corneal focus is fixed, the cornea cannot adjust to view objects at variable distances. The internal lens of the eye generally provides the fine tuning. The focusing power of the eye must be exactly matched to the length of the eye for clear vision to be present.

Refractive errors occur when a deviation occurs in the course of the light rays as they pass through the eye, thus preventing sharp focus on the retina. The three primary refractive errors are myopia, hyperopia, and astigmatism.

Myopia, or nearsightedness, is the condition characterized by an eye with too much focusing power, as a result of the cornea or crystalline lens being excessively curved or the globe itself being too long. As a result, light rays entering the eye are focused in front of the retina, and the retinal image is blurred. Near objects, which require the most focusing power, can be seen clearly, but distance objects are blurred. This condition is remedied by interposing a concave lens in front of the eye. This type of lens, also known as a *minus lens,* is thinnest in the center and has a divergent, or spreading effect on incoming light rays.

Hyperopia, or farsightedness, is a type of refractive error in which the eye, as a result of insufficient curvature of the cornea or crystalline lens, or because the eyeball itself is too short, or both, possesses insufficient refracting power. The focal point in these cases (or the locus where incoming light rays come to focus) is behind the retina, because light rays cannot bend sharply enough to focus on the retina. The closer an object is placed to the eye, the greater the retinal blur becomes; thus, a farsighted individual sees more clearly at far distance than at near. It must be noted that a person with a significant degree of farsightedness (and insufficient focusing ability) may focus inadequately even for distant objects and would, therefore, have blurred vision at both distant and near viewing. This condition is remedied by convex lenses, which also are known as *plus lenses.* Convex lenses are thicker in the center than at the edges and cause a convergent effect on light rays.

Astigmatism can be described as a "warpage" of the eye's optics caused by the cornea being steeper in certain directions, or meridians as well as the lens and globe itself having the potential for asphericity, or a lack of roundness. These irregular curvatures result in a distortion of the image, causing light rays to be spread out along a blurred line rather than achieving a pinpoint focus. This condition is remedied by the use of a *toric* aspherical lens, which has varying amounts of power in different meridians. With astigmatism, objects both near and far may be blurred.

Presbyopia, although not a refractive error per se, is a decreased ability to change the focus of the crystalline lens because of a loss of elasticity. This "hardening" of the lens occurs gradually throughout life but becomes apparent at about age 40. Patients of this age and older generally require spectacles for reading to compensate for this condition.

At this point, it is imperative to note that all visual systems are not created equal in terms of refraction or motor ability. Both eyes or one eye may be nearsighted, astigmatic, or farsighted while its mate may have no refractive error, or have an opposite condition, thus creating small or large imbalances between the two eyes.

When assessing the vergence or pointing system, an excess or insufficiency of convergence power may be present, and the eyes will then not point where they are focusing. This creates stress, discomfort, poor reading ability, and low self-esteem as a result of an individual's difficulty in performing visual tasks. Couple this with inherent problems within the accommodative or focusing subsystem described below, and one can see that lurking beneath the cover of 20/20 eyesight are all the ingredients for major visual dysfunction with resulting degradation in sensorimotor guidance.

Physiological Dysfunction

Physiological dysfunction refers to the mechanics of the autonomic nervous system and its effects on visual skills. It may surprise readers to learn that the visual system is influenced by the autonomic nervous system, which can heavily affect the visual development of the child of primary-school age, whose nervous system is still quite immature. Before the myelinization of the central nervous system is complete, by approximately age 14—and, coincidentally, puberty—the child can experience inconsistencies in homeostatic central nervous system balance because of a lack of balanced control between the sympathetic and parasympathetic systems. This imbalance can result in inconsistencies in visual function, especially with regard to focusing, because the ciliary body that controls focusing is under both sympathetic and parasympathetic control.

To further explain, accommodation or focusing of the crystalline lens is "owned" and innervated by two masters within the autonomic nervous system. The parasympathetic nervous system commands "focus" by causing the ciliary bodies to focus the lenses of the eyes, and the sympathetic system commands "do not focus" by causing the ciliary bodies to unfocus the lenses of the eyes. Hence the individual, especially between ages 4 and 8, may not automatically focus correctly or in a stable manner, resulting in intermittent blurring or poor resolution of detail that can cause the child to slow his or her reading rate to achieve optimum reception of the visual stimulus. Such children then perform as word readers rather than being able to group words together. They may lose their place when reading and have difficulty when shifting from one line of print to another. They often go up or down a line inappropriately. They also may have difficulties in spatial organization in paper-and-pencil tasks.

Note that difficulties in adequate focusing with accompanying poor resolution of detail also can cause children to manifest ciliary body spasm as they attempt to self-correct. This in turn causes a frontal headache or eye ache.

These deficiencies in accommodative innervation in a developing child can often be traced back to sympathetic override of the parasympathetic nervous system balance. The developing visual system is extremely dependent on the developing nervous system. In a sense, especially in the developmental years of ages 4 to 8, the dynamic skills of the visual system are *hostage* to the inconsistencies of an individual's developing nervous system. The term *sympathetic override* refers to the adrenalin-infused sympathetic side of the autonomic nervous system striving for attention at the expense of the calming control of the parasympathetic system being denervated. Sympathetic override also can be caused by emotional stress. Imagine the stress a child with learning disabilities experiences daily in school. Although this is a controversial idea, evidence suggests that sugar ingestion in children, particularly between ages 5 and 7 years, can create an adrenalin-induced response, resulting in sympathetic override. When the child is under visual stress, the fallout is that visual–spatial organization can suffer, color vision can suffer, and visual fields can constrict, all of which typically go unreported and unnoticed (Streff, 1962).

Another visual deficit results from dysfunctional neural control mechanisms that supply feedback to the visual skills of coordination of convergence and accommodation. It is very important that the relationship of these skills be precisely balanced to ensure comfortable, efficient vision. Consider, for example, the havoc that can result if the eyes converge at one distance while they are attempting to focus at another distance. This actually is a very common problem that can result in an uncomfortable visual mismatch, a short attention span, and problems with reading and comprehension.

Consider also that in reading, a *data link* between the book and the cognitive area of the brain is established. If the receptive nature of this data link is erratic because of problems associated with the visual skills of pointing, focusing, and tracking (saccades), then the data link becomes flawed. In the case of a child who is learning to read, this flawed data link has been shown to cause slow vision. For example, the child can call out single words when learning to read, but when asked to group or combine words (a skill essential for comprehension), he or she experiences problems because the visual skills responsible for a larger visual capture are not supporting the task. In other words, because of the flawed receptive quality of the incoming visual signal, the cognitive aspect can remain limited or dysfunctional.

The importance of an individual's visual skills in influencing his or her ability to maintain a stable data link without regressions or loss of fixation cannot be overstated. At the very least, it calls into question the reliability of reading testing in kindergarten through 3rd grade without proper visual skill assessment and remediation if warranted.

Fortunately, the profession of behavioral optometry has a well-developed body of knowledge regarding both the differential diagnosis and treatment of these above-mentioned visual difficulties. Specifically, lenses and prisms that alter an individual's vergence pattern (by producing either additional convergence or divergence) in spectacle-mounted form can be worn to reskew an individual's visual input into the proper balance and comfort zone. Likewise, lenses that balance an individual's focusing needs also can be prescribed. Behavioral optometry in fact refers to *remedial lenses* or *training lenses* as those lenses (often spectacle-mounted) whose purpose is to help the whole body–mind system work toward better balance, alignment, and coordination. Additionally, in- or out-of-office therapy may be suggested to augment the skewing action of the lenses.

Adult Visual Integration

In the preceding section, we dealt with the programming of the *emerging* visual system. Given the basic constructs presented therein, the outcomes may vary depending on factors such as one's inherited refractive state, opportunities for visual motor development (as in youth sports programs), and very importantly how much one learned about the capabilities of the human visual system.

When individuals are attempting to learn a visual motor skill, be it advanced or basic, the focus is usually on the motor act outcome (e.g., does the bat hit the ball squarely or is the gloved hand there to catch the ball). Beneath the expression of either success or failure at the task attempted, however, lies a visual-motor program waiting to be developed. With that thought in mind, it is important to realize that just because one did not have an idealized integrative adolescence all is not lost for future adult success.

We owe this fact to the master integrator, the human brain. As the body matures, the brain is busy running many programs. A neuromotor act that involves visual guidance therefore is not just repetitive but also involves attributes of memory and intelligence. In other words, the ability to direct motor action is not necessarily derived through conscious cognition.

This concept of intelligence driving visual motor can and should be a force to be considered in any visual integrative program. For example, just as visual repetition dulls the brain, *unpredictable* visual input is highly stimulating and is twice as effective in achieving integration. Even though it is sometimes difficult to orchestrate unpredictable external events, the beauty of working through the visual system becomes apparent when we consider the power of unpredictability that different lenses and prisms produce when placed before the eyes. Here is yet another reason for the two O's to work together in the spirit of integration.

To summarize, it is possible to assist in the further development of visual integrative abilities at any age. In fact, many seemingly diverse procedures may produce excellent results. However, it is the adaptive behavior of the *total action system* being led by the visual system that ensures results. The more one understands the power of intelligence behind the *visual system,* the more unlimited the therapeutic options become.

Assessment and Realities of the Visual System

To begin the complex process of behavioral optometry, the practitioner starts his or her examination of the optical functioning of the eye with a measurement of *unaided visual acuity.* This refers to the smallest line of letters that can be read on an eye chart with the naked eye. Almost everyone is familiar with the standard Snellen eye chart designations of 20/20, 20/30, 20/40, and so on, up to 20/200. These measurements actually express the individual's ability to resolve detail, using letters, numbers, or figures of various sizes on an eye chart positioned at 20 ft. The 20/20 line has characters of a size that, when resolved to their correct detail, represents an optical system in focus for optical infinity. In other words, an individual with no major refractive error or with a corrected refractive error in place, no abnormalities of the optical media, and good retinal function accompanied by a healthy optic nerve would be expected to see the 20/20 line.

Having thus defined a measure of an individual's sight, which is called *acuity,* we can see little about the definition that is dynamic or involves function. Herein lies the root of the common misconception that 20/20 is perfect vision.

As an example, although 20/20 acuity is helpful for passing the Department of Motor Vehicles' (DMV's) acuity test, it does not provide a measure of an individual's visual abilities that allow him or her to dynamically act and interact with the environment, which is the real test of driving ability. Just as passing the DMV's acuity test does not assess the actions and reactions that define being a good driver, neither does the distance Snellen chart address the individual's visual abilities or skills that allow him or her to dynamically interact with the environment.

In general, a primary-care vision examination should include at least a determination of acuities at both far and near; an assessment of ocular motility; a cover test (for assessment of over- or under-convergence tonicity); an assessment of pupillary responses; an assessment of refractive status, eye pressures, and confrontational visual fields; and an assessment of internal and external eye health.

It should be noted that, although these primary-care procedures satisfy the medical and legal requirements of an eye examination, they do not necessarily include the functional evaluation of an individual's dynamic visual abilities or skills, especially at near point. As we have discussed, visual skills are extremely important and should be assessed. However, even though the assessment of visual skills is extremely important to an understanding of visual function or dysfunction, this area is usually not probed in detail by eye care professionals other than by functional behavioral optometrists and neuro-optometrists, discussed below.

Areas of Vision Specialty

Having outlined the various visual dysfunctions, we now describe the specialists involved in treating these dysfunctions. A discussion of vision has traditionally invoked the image of the three "Os": (a) ophthalmology, (b) optometry, and (c) opticianry. The definitions used to be clear cut; however, because of recent legislative changes, optometrists now use therapeutic pharmaceutical agents to treat ocular disease and perform primary eye care that once was solely under the purview of ophthalmology. Now both ophthalmologists and optometrists dispense eyeglasses and contact lenses, and independent opticianry is in decline.

Ophthalmology

Ophthalmologists continue in their role as surgeons who diagnose and treat ocular pathology with surgery and medications as well as perform primary-care examinations. In treating strabismus, ophthalmologists also perform surgery to correct eye deviations. Ophthalmologists have also used *orthoptics*, a type of visual therapy, to treat strabismus.

Functional Behavioral Optometry

Behavioral optometry is a branch of organized optometry that has roots dating back to the late 1920s, when A. M. Skeffington, OD, began probing the mysteries of vision beyond the mere determination of refractive error. Armed with his insights, a new philosophy of optometry was formed that spoke to the process of vision involving learned skills as complex as the process of learning to speak, with its origins intimately related to a whole mind–body system.

These foundations of behavioral optometry are closely associated with the original Yale University Clinic of Child Development and the contributions of individuals such as Arnold Gesell, MD, who referred to the "whole human action system" being governed by "the input and output arrangement of the eye and brain," and Darryl Boyd Harmon, PhD, who argued that a purely optical theory of vision was inadequate because it failed to include the role of the brain in integrating experience or explain the phenomenon of brain–eye–hand–body coordination, which involves a constant process of instruction, feedback, and modified instruction.

Optometrists interested in this specialty area chiefly pursue their knowledge base through the College of Optometrists in Vision Development (COVD) and the Optometric Extension Program (OEP), both of which offer postgraduate learning opportunities. Individuals who desire to find a behavioral optometrist can contact the COVD for a listing of COVD-certified optometrists in their area. Maintaining certification in the COVD requires completion of a specified number of continuing education hours by the optometrist as well as testing for fellowship certification.

In addition to performing primary-care examinations, behavioral optometrists examine the visual system in regard to its relationship to dynamic functions. A behavioral vision analysis, for example, might assess the underlying causes of binocular dysfunction, such as a mismatch between an individual's focusing and convergence. It also would probe the relationship of vision to the other senses, especially gross motor function and eye–hand coordination. A behavioral optometrist might also analyze a patient's developmental history to determine periods of developmental lags, such as delayed self-lateralization and established hand dominance. Therapy then could consist of lenses and prisms in spectacle form to guide and stabilize the visual system, as well as in-office therapy. Behavioral optometrists also focus on visual skill enhancement. Therapy involving visual skills concerns itself with the flexibility and tonic state of the oculomotor act as well as learned integration of sensory information. It is *not* extraocular muscle strengthening. The extraocular muscles, as well as the ciliary body, have unlimited strength; their dysfunctional behavior results from inappropriate neurocontrol and tonicity problems. Muscle strengthening is not a consideration.

Neuro-Optometry

Like functional or behavioral optometry, neuro-optometry is also a subspecialty of optometry. Neuro-optometrists perform diagnostic testing to determine specific acquired visual dysfunctions or deficits that are a direct result of physical disability; traumatic brain injury; or other neurological insults, such as cerebral palsy or multiple sclerosis. They also work closely with a rehabilitation team to reestablish *balance* in the individual with vision difficulties.

Collaboration Between Occupational Therapy and Behavioral Optometry

Occupational therapy and behavioral optometry have much to gain by partnering in sharing professional concepts. This has been well demonstrated in the intertwined relationship of one's total action system and the total action system's relationship to vision. This partnership has the potential for a long and fruitful union, because the origins of both disciplines are deeply rooted in function. In 1987 Steven Cool, PhD, then an adjunct professor of occupational therapy and associate professor of physiological optics at Pacific University, authored an article entitled "Occupational Therapy and Functional Optometry: An Interaction Whose Time Has Come?" Perhaps it is now time to remove the question mark from that article, because without a doubt, both occupational therapy and behavioral optometry are deeply and philosophically rooted in function. (Cool, 1987).

In addition to having an emphasis on function in common, both occupational therapy and optometry also share many commonalities in understanding the processes of development and integration. The area of integration is steeped in the contributions of occupational therapy, and this is the perfect place to begin rapport between the two "functional Os": optometry and occupational therapy. Just as occupational therapists have honed techniques for creating "movement" within the body's related motor systems, behavioral optometrists also have honed and developed skills and techniques for creating movement both within the visual system and the body's related motor systems.

It has been written that the average time to foster new thinking in a profession is 20 years. Perhaps with the updating and revisions to the second edition of this groundbreaking book, we can escalate that time span. To that end, I hope the material in this chapter will further communication and rapport between these two dynamic professions.

References

Carpenter, M. B. (1991). *Core text of neuroanatomy*. Philadelphia: Williams and Wilkins.

Cool, S. (1987, September). Occupational therapy and functional optometry: An interaction whose time has come? *Sensory Integration Special Interest Section, 10*(3), 1, 5.

Gaymard, C. J. (1998). Temporal limits of spatial working memory in humans. *European Journal of Neuroscience, 10,* 794–797.

Gesell, A. G., Ilg, F., & Ames, L. (1946). *Growth: The child from five to ten* (rev. ed.). New York: Harper and Row.

Gilbert, C. D., Das, A., Ito, M., Kapadia, M., & Westheimer, G. (2000). Spatial integration and cortical dynamics. In National Academies Press (Ed.), *Vision: From photon to perception* (pp. 59–66). Washington, DC: National Academies Press.

Goodale, M. A., & Millner, A. D. (1992). Separate visual pathways for perception and action. *Trends in Neuroscience, 15,* 20–25.

Jeannerod, M., Paulignon, Y., & Weiss, P. (1998). Grasping an object: One movement, several components. *Novartis Foundation Symposium, 218,* 5–16.

Jouen, M., Lepecq, J. C., Gapenne, O., & Bertenthal, B. I. (2000). Optic flow sensitivity in neonates. *Infant Behavior and Development, 23,* 271–284.

Streff, J. (1962). Preliminary observations of a non-malingering syndrome. *Optometric Weekly, 53*(12).

Streff, J. (1971). Lecture notes. Southern College of Optometry.

Appendix 1.A.
Anatomy and Function of the Eye

Steven Schiff, OD

The following is intended to serve as a reference for health care professionals who encounter patients with ocular conditions. The information contained herein will provide the anatomical basis for an overall understanding for such conditions. Emphasis is placed on those structures that play the most important role in the visual sense.

As light enters the eye, it travels through various media, and the rays are bent, or refracted. Refraction of light rays make it possible for light from a large area to focus on a small surface, the *retina*.

The Eyelids

As the eyelids are the most anterior structure, they serve a protective function. They protect the eye in several ways: When closed, they shield the eye from foreign objects; when open, the eyelashes catch and filter fine airborne particles. In addition, the many glands found on the edge of the eyelids produce the tear film. The tears moisten and hence lubricate the cornea and contain antibodies to destroy pathogenic bacteria that may be present in airborne particles.

Several neurologic disorders will cause the eyelids to either droop, which is known as *ptosis,* or to retract, causing the eyeball to seem larger on the affected side. Should a patient present with ptosis or lid retraction without previous history, immediate referral to the appropriate specialist is in order.

The Cornea

The *cornea* is the main refracting element of the eye due to its steep curvature. It is primarily the curvature of the cornea that determines the presence and extent of myopia (nearsightedness), hyperopia (farsightedness), and astigmatism. It is excessive curvature that produces myopia, insufficient curvature that produces hyperopia, and unequal curvature or "warpage" of the cornea that produces astigmatism.

The cornea is composed of three basic layers. The *epithelium* is the outermost layer and is therefore most vulnerable to damage by foreign objects. If there is a history of "foreign body" removal in the past, there may be a visible scar, with subjective complaints of glare, possibly worse in dark environments.

The *stroma* is the middle layer and comprises 90% of the corneal thickness. Here is where the corneal nerves are found, and as the cornea is richly supplied with sensory nerves, it is one of the most sensitive tissues of the body.

The *endothelium* is the single layer of cells that separate the cornea from the anterior chamber, the next structure in the eye. Biochemical reactions between this layer and the aqueous humor maintain proper osmotic balance of the cornea.

In its normal state, the cornea is transparent, which is essential for proper image formation on the retina. Microscopic anatomy of the cornea makes it an ideal optical instrument—the smoothness and uniformity of the epithelial cell layer allows for uninterrupted transmission of light rays. In addition, the corneal cells have no pigmentation and blood vessels to interfere with light transmission.

The Sclera

The *sclera*, or "white of the eye," is the tough external layer that surrounds the eyeball everywhere except at the cornea (which may be considered the forward extension of the sclera). It is composed of numerous layers of connective tissue that give it its strength, and it is opaque, allowing no light to enter the eye, which reduces light scatter and glare.

The Aqueous Humor

The *aqueous humor* is the watery fluid that fills the anterior chamber, which comprises the area behind the cornea but anterior to the lens. In most of the major ocular structures, there are no blood vessels. The aqueous humor is the source of nutrients to these structures; it also functions as the vehicle for disposal of metabolites of cellular processes. It is derived from the bloodstream and is manufactured by the ciliary body.

By way of steady aqueous formation and drainage, the pressure within the eyeball is maintained at a fairly constant level. Excessive amounts of aqueous humor occur when there is too much production or impaired drainage. This causes an increase in intraocular pressure, which is known as *glaucoma*.

The ciliary body is found in the anterior chamber. It is responsible for production of aqueous humor. In addition, the ciliary body contains the ciliary muscle, which is responsible for altering the shape of the lens during the process of accommodation.

The *iris* is the colored part of the eye. It is a circular structure, with a hole in the center, which is the pupil. The size of the pupil is regulated by the musculature of the iris. The iris contains two muscles: the sphincter and the dilator. When contracted, the sphincter decreases pupil size, thereby reducing the amount of light entering the eye. The dilator muscles radiate away from the pupil and serve to increase the size of it, and therefore, the amount of light entering it. The size of the pupil is quite variable, ranging from 1 mm when fully contracted to more than 9 mm when dilated. Pupils are reflexive, responding to light stimuli on the retina. This is known as the light reflex. It is linked to accommodative function (near reflex).

Pupil size also can be affected by neurological, cardiac, or central nervous system conditions, or by drug use. Unequal size and/or reactivity can signal neurological problems such as a stroke. Dilated, unresponsive pupils are often seen in cardiac arrest, unconscious patients, or those on amphetamines. Constricted pupils may indicate central nervous system disorders or narcotic use.

Hippus is the term used to describe pupils that are constantly changing in size. This is a normal phenomenon, often seen in young people, and is not indicative of pathology of any kind. *Anisocoria* is by definition an unequal pupil size in one eye as compared to the other. About 25%–30% of the general population have this condition, with no associated pathology.

The Lens

The crystalline *lens* is found immediately behind the iris and is a secondary refractive element of the eye. It accounts for approximately 25% of the eye's refractive power. At distances of 20 feet or more, light rays that enter the eye are for all purposes parallel. Within this distance, the ciliary muscle acts on the lens in varying degrees to provide accommodation. This enables the eye to focus on objects at various distances. The lens is normally transparent, elastic, and very flexible. It is avascular and obtains its nutrients from the aqueous humor.

With aging, the lens undergoes a loss of its elasticity, and the accommodative function decreases at a steady rate. This makes it difficult to focus clearly on near objects. Patients older than age 40 generally require spectacles for reading to compensate for this condition, which is known as *presbyopia*.

The lens also becomes increasingly "sclerosed" (accumulation of yellowish pigment) with aging. This may be partially due to absorption of ultraviolet radiation in sunlight. When this pigment begins to decrease light reaching the retina, visual acuity becomes worse. This is known as a *cataract* and is treated via surgical removal of the lens, which is replaced with an artificial lens, known as an *implant*. Implants have been used for the past decade or so. Prior to this, high-powered contact lenses or spectacles were required to compensate for the refractive power that the lens originally provided.

The vitreous humor is the jelly-like substance that fills the posterior chamber, the largest chamber of the eyeball. It fills the entire space between the lens and the retina. The vitreous humor keeps the eyeball firm and round and physically supports the retinal layers by keeping them under constant pressure against the sclera. Dead red blood cells within the vitreous humor are seen as "floaters," or objects perceived by the patient to be present in their visual field.

The retina can be thought of as "the film" where the image develops. It is transparent and contains 10 different layers of nerve cells. It is actually an extension of brain tissue. Here we find the photoreceptors, the *rods*, which are more concentrated in the periphery and are sensitive to low light and red light. They are primarily responsible for night vision. Incidently, this is why most instrument panels are shades of red; the rod photoreceptors are better able to respond to this color. The *cones* are more centrally located, and they provide fine object detail and color vision. They function best in bright light. During dark adaptation, the rods gradually take over visual function.

The photoreceptors function by way of pigments that are light sensitive. Production of these pigments depends on vitamin A. Color blindness is caused by deficiency or absence of one or more cone types. Red–green color blindness is most common; this is an inherited condition seen in 10% of all men but rarely seen in women.

The Macula

The highest concentration of cones is found at the fovea/macula: The macular region is the central retina, about 5 mm in size. This is the area of the retina responsible for high visual resolution and color vision. Here we find the highest concentration of cones and the best visual acuity. The fovea is a small-1.5 mm depression in the center of the macula, and the cones found here have the finest diameters and provide the best visual acuity. When an object is viewed, the person reflexively moves the eyeball so that the most important part of the image falls on the fovea. This is known as *central fixation*. The several common conditions associated with the macula include macular degeneration, macular edema, and macular hole.

The Optic Nerve

The *optic nerve* carries visual information generated by the rods and the cones and transmits the visual sensory messages to the brain for processing. It is the only area on the retina where vision is absent; this is known as the "blind spot." Optic nerves leave the back of each eye and meet at the chiasm.

The Extraocular Muscles

The extraocular muscles attach from the skull bones to the sclera. They control the movements of the eyeball within its orbital socket. There are six muscles per eye, and they can be divided into two groups, based on their position and resultant effect on movement: The *recti muscles,* of which there are four, are responsible for the basic up–down and left–right movements, and the two *oblique muscles,* give the eye the ability to perform diagonal movements (see Figure 1.A).

The superior rectus muscle is named for its attachment to the top of the globe, and it is responsible for upgaze. The inferior rectus attaches at the bottom of the globe and pulls the eyeball downward, for downgaze, such as required in reading. The medial and lateral recti muscles are used to direct the eyeball in a sideways (lateral) direction.

The superior oblique muscle, when innervated, primarily causes the eyeball to turn inward (adduction) and downward. The inferior oblique has the opposite effect, causing the eyeball to turn out (abduction) and down.

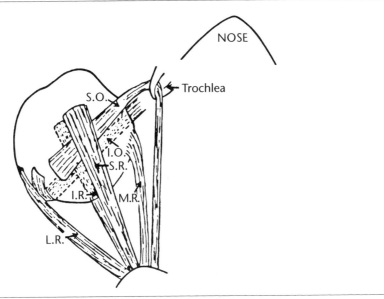

Figure 1A.1. The extraocular muscles, viewed from above.
Note. S.O. = superior oblique, I.O. = inferior oblique, S.R. = superior rectus, I.R. = inferior rectus, M.R. = media rectus, L.R. = lateral rectus
From *Ophthalmology Made Ridiculously Simple* by S. Goldberg. Copyright © 1966 by MedMaster, Inc. Reprinted with permission.

The extraocular muscles are among the most rapidly acting and precisely controlled skeletal muscles in the body. Cranial nerves 3, 4, and 6 innervate these muscles. They are yoked, meaning each muscle is paired with muscles in the opposite eye; this allows the eyes to move in the same direction at the same time. Conjugate movements of the two eyes are known as *versions,* compared to *ductions,* which refers to the movements of a single eye in its various fields of gaze. When the eyes move in opposite directions, the term *vergence* is used. Movement of the eyes toward each other, or nasally, is known as *convergence,* and the movement of the eyes outward is known as *divergence.* The medial and lateral recti muscles are primarily responsible for vergence movements, and improper coordination of these muscles causes the binocular deficits.

Appendix 1.B.
Overview of Ocular Diseases and Disorders

Condition	Affected Area	Cause	Visual Effects	Mode of Detection	Treatment	Prognosis
Achromatopsia (total color blindness)	Retina (cone malformation).	Hereditary.	Decreased visual acuity to 20/200, extreme photophobia, and nystagmus. Visual fields are normal.	Color vision screening test and electrodiagnostic tests, especially using the electroretinogram (ERG).	Optical aids, sunglasses, and dim illumination.	Nonprogressive nystagmus and photophobia reduce with age.
Albinism (total or partial lack of pigment)	Macula (underdeveloped).	Hereditary.	Decreased visual acuity (20/200 to 20/70), nystagmus, photophobia, high-refractive effort, and astigmatism. Visual fields variable, and color vision is normal.	Family history and ocular examination.	Painted or pinhole contact lenses, absorptive lenses, optical aids, and dim illumination.	Nonprogressive.
Aniridia	Iris (underdeveloped).	Hereditary.	Decreased visual acuity, photophobia, possible nystagmus, cataracts, displaced lens, and underdeveloped retina. Visual fields are normal. Secondary complication: glaucoma, with accompanying constriction of the visual fields, squint, and lens opacification.	Clinical observation of missing iris tissue.	Pinhole contact lenses, sunglasses, optical aids, and dim illumination.	Milder forms develop slow, progressive cataracts; severe forms develop glaucoma and corneal opacification.
Cataracts (congenital)	Lens (opacity).	Hereditary, congenital anomalies (rubella, Marfan's syndrome, Down syndrome), infection or drugs during pregnancy, and severe malnutrition during pregnancy.	Decreased visual acuity, blurred vision, nystagmus, squint, photophobia, slight constriction in the peripheral visual fields are possible, but visual fields are normal.	Ophthalmoscopy and slit-lamp biomicroscope.	Surgery as early as possible, cases of visual impairment.	After surgery, inability to accommodate; problems with glare, which are corrected with spectacles or contact lenses. Complications from surgery: glaucoma, retinal detachment, hemorrhage of the vitreous humor or retina.

Condition	Site	Cause	Symptoms	Assessment	Treatment	Prognosis
Cataracts (senile)	Lens (opacity).	Age.	Progressively blurred vision; near vision is better than distance vision.	Same as for congenital cataracts.	Surgery, with resultant cataract spectacles, contact lenses, lens implant (IOL, intraocular lens).	Same as for congenital cataracts. Complications from surgery: glaucoma, retinal detachment, hemorrhage of the vitreous, infection. Better candidate for intraocular lens (IOL) implants.
Cataracts (traumatic)	Lens (opacity).	Head injury or metallic foreign body in the eye.	Blurred vision, redness, and inflammation of the eye and decreased visual acuity. Complications: infection, uveitis, retinal detachment, and glaucoma.	Same as for congenital and senile cataracts.	Surgery after inflammation subsides.	Same as for congenital and senile cataracts.
Coloboma	Various parts of the eye may have been deformed, severity depending on when deformity occurred during development.	Hereditary.	Decreased visual acuity, nystagmus, strabismus, photophobia, and loss of visual and superior fields. Secondary complication: cataracts. Associated conditions: microphthalmia, polydactyly, and mental retardation.	Fundus examination.	Cosmetic contact lenses, sunglasses, and optical aids.	Usually fairly stable.
Diabetes mellitus	Retina.	Hereditary.	Diplopia, inability to accommodate, fluctuating vision, loss of color vision, loss of visual field re-refractive error, decreased visual acuity, hemorrhaging of blood vessels in the retina, retinal detachment. Secondary complications: glaucoma and cataracts. Associated conditions: cardiovascular problems, skin problems, and kidney problems.	Ophthalmoscopy; reports of fluctuating vision.	Insulin injections, dietary controls, spectacles, and laser beam surgery. Various illumination control aids.	Variation in acuity common.

(Continued)

Condition	Affected Area	Cause	Visual Effects	Mode of Detection	Treatment	Prognosis
Degenerative myopia (nearsightedness)	Elongation of the eye; stretching of the posterior of the eye.	Hereditary.	Decreased visual acuity in the distance, vitreous floaters, metamorphopsia. Normal visual field unless retina is detached. Secondary complications: retinal detachment and swelling or hemorrhaging of the macula.	Fundus examination.	Prescription correction, preferably contact lenses; optical aids; and high illumination.	Unpredictable rate of progression.
Down syndrome (mongolism)	Various parts of the eye.	Hereditary; extra No. 21 chromosome.	Decrease of visual acuity, squint, nystagmus, severe myopia, Brushfield spots, congenital cataracts, and keratoconus. Color vision and visual fields are normal. Associated conditions: mental retardation; cardiac abnormalities; hypotonia; saddle-shaped nose; large protruding tongue; and a short, squat stature.	Physical appearance. Complete medical workup.	Depending on patient's intellectual level, optical aids, prescription correction.	Medical problems more severe than usual. Good prognosis.
Glaucoma (acute attack)	Same as for congenital and adult glaucoma.	Inability of the aqueous to drain.	Nausea, severe redness of the eye, headache, and severe pain.	Same as for congenital and adult glaucoma.	Emergency surgery.	Without surgery, permanent damage to the ocular tissues and loss of visual acuity and in peripheral vision.
Glaucoma (adult)	Same as for congenital glaucoma.	Hereditary or the result of changes in the eye after surgery.	Headaches in the front portion of the head, especially in the morning; seeing halos around lights; decreased visual acuity, loss of visual fields, photophobia, and constricted peripheral fields in severe cases.	Same as for congenital glaucoma.	Eye drops, optical aids, sunglasses.	With treatment, depends on the innate resistance of the structures of the eye. Blindness if not treated.
Glaucoma (congenital)	Tissues of the eye damaged from increased intraocular pressure.	Hereditary.	Excessive tearing, photophobia, opacity or haze on lens, buphthalmos, poor visual acuity, and constricted visual fields.	Tonometry, study of the visual fields, and ophthalmoscopy.	Eye drops; surgery as soon as possible to prevent extensive damage.	Same as for adult glaucoma.

Condition	Part of eye affected	Cause	Symptoms	Detection	Treatment	Prognosis
Histoplasmosis	Macula or periphery (scattered lesions).	Fungus transmitted by spores found in dried excrement of animals.	In the macula: decreased visual acuity, central scotoma, and deficient color vision. In the periphery: scotoma corresponding to the area of lesions.	Ophthalmoscopy.	Optical aids for visual problems; steroids for physical condition.	Can be life-threatening if not treated.
Keratoconus	Cornea (stretched to a cone shape).	Hereditary. Manifests in second decade.	Increased distortion of entire visual field; progressive decrease in visual acuity, especially in the distance. Associated conditions: retinitis pigmentosa, aniridia, Down syndrome, and Marfan's syndrome.	Ophthalmoscopy, retinoscopy, keratometry, and slit-lamp biomicroscope.	Hard contact lenses in the early stages; keratoplasty (corneal transplant) as needed.	Without keratoplasty, progressive degenerative thinning of cornea until cornea ruptures and blindness ensues.
Marfan's syndrome (disease of the connective tissues of the body)	Various parts of the eye.	Hereditary.	Dislocation of the lens, decreased visual acuity, severe myopia, dislocated or multiple pupil, retinal detachment with accompanying field loss, different-colored eyes, squint, nystagmus, and bluish sclera. Associated conditions: skeletal abnormalities; long, thin fingers and toes; cardiovascular problems; and muscular underdevelopment.	Medical examination and evaluation.	Optical aids. Surgical or optical management of the dislocated lens.	Vision problems stable; medical problems are more significant.
Retinal detachment	Retina (portions detach from supporting structure and atrophy).	Numerous, including diabetes, diabetic retinopathy, degenerative myopia, and a blow to the head.	Appearance of flashing lights, sharp stabbing pain in the eye, visual field loss, micropsia, color defects, and decreased visual acuity if the macula is affected.	Ophthalmoscopy and an internal eye examination.	Laser beam surgery and cryosurgery, depending on the type and cause of the detachment; optical aids; and usually high illumination.	Guarded.

(Continued)

Appendix 1.B. Overview of Ocular Diseases and Disorders (*Continued*)

Condition	Affected Area	Cause	Visual Effects	Mode of Detection	Treatment	Prognosis
Retinitis pigmentosa	Retina (degenerative pigmentary condition).	Hereditary.	Decreased visual acuity, photophobia, constriction of the visual fields (loss in the peripheral field), and night blindness. Usher's syndrome, Laurence–Moon–Biedl's syndrome, and Leber's syndrome.	Electrodiagnostic testing, especially ERG, and ophthalmoscopy.	Optical aids, prisms. No known medical cure; genetic counseling is essential.	Slow, progressive loss in the visual fields that may lead to blindness.
Retrolental fibroplasia	Retina (growth of blood vessels) and vitreous humor.	High levels of oxygen administered to premature infants; occasionally found in full-term infants.	Decreased visual acuity, severe myopia, scarring, and retinal detachment, with resultant visual field loss and possible blindness. Secondary complications: glaucoma and uveitis.	Ophthalmoscopy.	Optical aids and illumination control devices.	Poor, in severe cases, where further detachments can be expected in third decade.
Rubella	Various parts of the eye.	Virus transmitted to the fetus by the mother during pregnancy.	Congenital glaucoma, congenital cataracts, microphthalmia, decreased visual acuity, and constriction of the visual fields. Associated conditions: heart defects, ear defects, and mental deficiency.	Ophthalmoscopy, slit-lamp biomicroscope, tonometry, and family history.	Surgery for glaucoma and cataracts, optical aids, establishment of appropriate educational goals.	Poor; post-surgical inflammation.
Toxoplasmosis	Retina, especially macula (lesions).	Intraocular infection caused by *Toxoplasma gondii*. In congenital type, fetus exposed to organism; in acquired type, through contact with infected animals or ingested.	Loss in visual fields corresponding to location of lesion, squint, decreased visual acuity if macula is affected, severe brain damage if congenital.	Ophthalmoscopy.	Optical aids, usually good responses to magnification.	Nonprogressive, although new lesions may develop.

Source. Jose, R. T. (Ed.). (1983). *Understanding Low Vision.* New York: American Foundation for the Blind. Reproduced with permission.

Optometric Assessment and Treatment of Low Vision in Children and Adults

Bruce P. Rosenthal, OD, FAAO
Michael L. Fischer, OD, FAAO

Several definitions of low vision have been used over the past 75 years. One of the first was developed by Faye (1984), who described low vision as bilateral subnormal visual acuity or an abnormal visual field resulting from a disorder in the visual system. The vision loss in low vision cannot be corrected to a normal visual acuity level with standard corrective lenses (including contact or intraocular lenses) or by medical or surgical intervention. In 1975, Mehr and Freid described *low vision* or *partial sight* as reduced central acuity or visual field loss that, even with the best optical correction provided by regular lenses, still results in visual impairment from a performance standpoint. Mehr and Freid pointed out that this definition assumes that the loss is bilateral; that some form of vision remains; and that regular lenses do not include reading aids over +4.00 diopter, telescopes, pinholes, visors, or other unusual devices, which are categorized as low vision aids.

Arditi and Rosenthal (1996) introduced a different definition of *functional visual impairment* as a significant limitation of visual capability resulting from disease, trauma, or a congenital condition that cannot be fully ameliorated by standard refractive correction, medication, or surgery and that is manifested by one or more of the following:

- Insufficient visual resolution (worse than 20/60 in the better eye with best correction of ametropia),
- Inadequate field of vision (worse than 20° along the widest meridian in the eye with the more intact central field, or homonymous bilateral hemianopsia or quadrantanopsia), or
- Reduced peak contrast sensitivity (0.3 log unit loss in the better eye).

This definition addresses some of the primary visual disorders that occupational therapists may encounter; that is, the definition specifically includes *hemianopsia,* which is a loss of one-half of the visual field owing to a stroke, tumor, or other damage in the cortical visual pathway. This definition also tries to quantify a loss in contrast, which may affect mobility, activities of daily living (ADLs), and reading.

In the context of rehabilitative medicine, Colenbrander (1976) was the first to introduce the following terms to the field of low vision: *disorder, impairment, disability,* and *handicap.* Colenbrander defined a visual *disorder* as any deviation from normal structure or function of the body or parts thereof (e.g., cataract, cornea, scar on the retina). A disorder leads to an *impairment,* which is a disorder interfering with an organ function (e.g., reduced visual acuity, decreased contrast sensitivity, reduced visual field, color vision deficits). An impairment can then lead to a *disability,* which is the lack, loss, or reduction of an individual's ability to perform certain tasks (e.g., a person cannot read a newspaper or travel safely in the environment). Note that *impairment* refers to the basic functions performed by a part of the body; *disability* refers to tasks performed by a person. A visual *handicap* is the societal and economic consequence of a disability. A person could be considered handicapped if reading the newspaper is an important activity in his or her life.

Colenbrander (1976) described *visual acuity impairment, visual field impairment,* and *contrast sensitivity impairment* as a progression of loss from none, to slight, to moderate, to severe, to profound, to near-total, to total visual loss. He assessed visual disability and visual handicap in the same terms. Under the classification *visual disability,* a person with near-normal vision can perform all visual tasks, whereas an individual with a moderate to severe visual loss needs optical appliances for detailed visual tasks. An individual with a severe visual disability needs optical appliances and other senses for gross visual tasks. With respect to visual handicap, an individual with normal or near-normal vision can meet societal expectations, whereas a person with a moderate to total visual handicap cannot meet societal expectations visually.

Colenbrander (1976) also noted that clinicians and researchers should use accurate universal terminology that will maximize communication and teamwork and foster further development of rehabilitation techniques.

During the past 25 years, the expression *low vision* has taken on various connotations. It has not only come to define a person with a bilateral vision loss but also has become synonymous with an area of expertise dealing with people who have visual impairments. *Vision rehabilitation* has come generally to imply a team approach in the remediation process.

It should be noted that *amblyopia* is sometimes confused with or substituted for *low vision.* However, by definition *amblyopia* is a monocular loss in vision rather than a loss in both eyes.

Legal Blindness

Being diagnosed with low vision does not necessarily mean that a person is legally blind. *Legal blindness* is a term that was introduced in the United States in the 1930s so that state and federal aid could be offered to blind people (Nowakowski, 1994), and it is still used today as a measure of a person's eligibility for such benefits. Legal blindness is used to identify individuals who have a visual acuity of 20/200 or less in the better eye, or a visual field of 20° or less in the better eye. It also should be noted that, by international standards, an individual may be considered to have low vision when visual acuity is as good as 20/40 or 20/50 (6/12 or 6/15, respectively, when the numerator in the test distance is expressed in meters) or the visual field is anywhere from 100° to 20° (Johnston, 1991).

Epidemiology

Four classic studies—(a) the Framingham Eye Study (Kahn et al., 1977), (b) the Beaver Dam Eye Study (Klein, Klein, Linton, & De Mets, 1991), (c) the Baltimore Eye Survey (Tielsch, Sommer, Witt, Katz, & Royall, 1990), and (d) the Mud Creek Valley Study (Dana et al., 1990)—concluded that visual impairment and blindness increase significantly with age. Greater life expectancy translates into more people with significant visual impairments. In fact, it has been estimated that, by 2030, 65.6 million people in the United States will be age 65 years or older (U.S. Bureau of the Census, 1989). With increasing numbers of older people comes an increased prevalence of conditions associated with an aging population. These include macular degeneration, glaucoma, diabetic retinopathy, and optic atrophy. The Beaver Dam Eye Study (Klein et al., 1991) estimated that 1 in 4 people ages 70 and older have age-related macular degeneration.

Certain populations have a greater prevalence of ocular disease with aging. For example, the Baltimore Eye Survey (Tielsch et al., 1990) pointed out that the prevalence of visual impairment and blindness is twice as high in the Black population compared with the White population owing to the incidence of glaucoma and diabetic retinopathy.

Some conditions, including optic atrophy, cataract, and macular degeneration, can have a hereditary component. A careful case history often will detail the incidence of the condition in immediate family members as well as in past generations. Some diseases, if present during pregnancy (e.g., rubella or syphilis), may be passed on to the fetus and can have ocular complications that are manifested at birth. Other causative factors resulting in congenital low vision include prematurity, low birthweight, fetal alcohol syndrome, and drug abuse during pregnancy.

Diagnostic Testing for Conditions Causing Low Vision

From a patient management perspective, it is valuable to have an accurate diagnosis of the patient's ocular condition before beginning low vision rehabilitation services.

Knowing the patient's diagnosis will affect the types of low vision devices prescribed as well as what other vision rehabilitation services are recommended, and when.

Some conditions are easily diagnosed as part of a routine eye examination, through careful history taking and basic examination procedures, including biomicroscopy (to evaluate the front of the eye) and ophthalmoscopy (to view the internal ocular structures). However, it is sometimes necessary to perform specialized testing procedures to establish or confirm a diagnosis. This testing may be available in some private practices, but in some areas it may be available only in a hospital or university eye clinic.

If a definitive diagnosis has not been established before the low vision examination, the low vision doctor may request additional testing after the examination as part of the management of the patient. Some examples of these special procedures are discussed in the following sections.

Electrodiagnostic Procedures

Electroretinogram

The *electroretinogram (ERG)* is an objective test that reflects overall retinal function. It is the summed electrical response from the retina resulting from stimulation of the rods and cones by light energy. It is the test most frequently used to confirm or deny the diagnosis of retinitis pigmentosa (Sherman & Bass, 1996).

Visual Evoked Potential

The *visual evoked potential (VEP)* is another objective test of visual function. The electrical activity of the brain is monitored at the occipital cortex by scalp electrodes while the patient views a visual stimulus. The electrical response at the occipital cortex is measured and recorded. Because the response is evoked by a visual stimulus, it is called an *evoked potential* (Sherman & Bass, 1996). The VEP is used in certain situations as an objective measurement of visual acuity and of retinal and optic nerve dysfunction in the absence of observable pathology. The test also is used in objectively estimating binocular fusion and stereopsis and in the prognostic assessment of amblyopia, as well as with nonverbal patients diagnosed with autism, Down syndrome, Alzheimer's disease, or cerebral palsy (Sherman & Sutija, 1991).

The most common types of visual evoked potential tests include the flash VEP and the pattern VEP. *Flash VEP* is a method of obtaining the visual evoked potential using a bright flashing stimulus. It may be used in predicting the integrity of the visual system in a patient with a scarred cornea or cataracts. *Pattern VEP* is a response to checkerboard pattern stimulation. The checkerboard squares appear on a monitor in various sizes and rapidly alternate from black to white to black squares. The pattern VEP is the one test that allows objective measurement of visual acuity. Pattern VEP results can be influenced by uncorrected refractive error or lack of attention on the stimulus.

Electro-Oculogram

The *electro-oculogram (EOG)* is another electrodiagnostic test that assesses the integrity of the pigment epithelium layer in the retina. (Sherman & Bass, 1984). The EOG is not used as frequently as the ERG or VEP but is used as a differential diagnostic test for certain conditions, such as Best's vitelliform dystrophy and toxic retinal damage.

Ultrasound

Ultrasound (Bass & Sherman, 1991) is a test that uses the reflection of sound waves to provide a visual representation of the internal ocular structures. This is especially useful when media opacities make it difficult or impossible to see inside the eye. An A-scan is frequently used to determine the axial length of the eye for the determination of the power of an intraocular lens used in cataract surgery, and a B-scan is used in many clinical applications, including to determine the existence of a detached retina, intraocular tumors, and lens dislocation.

Other Procedures

Other tests that may be used to obtain additional diagnostic information about a patient's condition include the following:

* *Fluorescein angiography* (Fingeret, Casser, & Woodcome, 1990), a diagnostic photography procedure used to detect vascular compromise to the retina, choroid, and optic nerve, allows evaluation of the presence of subretinal vasculature changes that may not be seen with the ophthalmoscope. It is frequently used in the assessment of certain forms of macular degeneration and diabetic retinopathy, among other conditions.
* *Magnetic resonance imaging* (Oshinskie, 1991), a noninvasive method of examining an internal body structure including the orbit and its components, has been shown to be effective in imaging many brain lesions and space-occupying lesions. It is used, for example, in imaging lesions in multiple sclerosis and intraocular tumors.
* *Computerized axial tomography* (Oshinskie, 1991), uses x-rays like conventional tomography but produces a series of slices of the structure studied. The scan is used in the diagnosis of ocular masses, tumors of the optic nerve, blowout fractures of the orbit, and bone erosion.

Medical Treatment of Conditions Causing Low Vision

Although conditions that cause low vision are not correctable, medical intervention can still produce some improvement in the patient's visual function or can slow or stop the progression of the patient's condition. Such interventions may take place either prior to the initial low vision evaluation or while low vision rehabilitation is taking place. These can include

* Removal of a cataract;
* Various treatments of the retina for hemorrhaging or leakage of fluid in conditions such as macular degeneration or diabetic retinopathy, including thermal laser photo-

coagulation, photodynamic therapy, injection of steroids or anti-angiogenic agents, and other treatments that are being evaluated;

- Surgery for a detached retina, sometimes associated with high myopia or trauma;
- Corneal transplant;
- Determination of the type of or combination of eye drops, systemic medications, laser treatment, and surgery to reduce the eye pressure in glaucoma therapy;
- Vitrectomy (a procedure involving removal of the vitreous, a jellylike fluid occupying the center of the eye) when there is, for example, hemorrhage, debris from trauma, or fibrous bands that cloud the vitreous; and
- Lid problems, such as ectropion (lid turning out), entropion (lid turning in), or ptosis (drooping of the lid).

Low Vision Evaluation

The referral for a low vision evaluation is usually made to a low vision service in a rehabilitation agency, a private group or individual practice with an optometrist or ophthalmologist specializing in low vision, or a vision service at a university. (Some of the many programs for advanced study in low vision include low vision residencies and internships as well as the Lighthouse Low Vision Continuing Education Program.) Institutions offering low vision services often have additional services that may be of benefit in the evaluation or rehabilitation of the patient with low vision. For example, an agency that specializes in vision rehabilitation may also offer

- Training in the use of low vision devices;
- Orientation and mobility training;
- Social services and counseling;
- Techniques or training in ADLs;
- Technology and computer training;
- Reader services;
- Art, music, and dance classes;
- Children's services; and
- Adult and children recreation services.

Remediation of visual impairment clearly involves more than just treating the eyes. Many individuals may take part in the vision rehabilitation of people with low vision. The low vision team may include one or more of the following:

- An optometrist or ophthalmologist;
- An optician;
- An orientation and mobility specialist;
- A rehabilitation teacher;
- A social worker;
- A teacher for those with visual impairments, or other educators;
- A low vision instructor;

- A certified low vision therapist;
- A nurse;
- An occupational therapist;
- A physical therapist;
- A psychologist;
- An internist;
- A neurologist;
- A diabetologist;
- A psychiatrist.

A low vision evaluation is generally recommended or is provided by the optometrist or ophthalmologist.

Evaluating Visual Impairment: The Case History

Low vision remediation begins with a functional low vision evaluation. As noted earlier, the low vision evaluation generally follows medical intervention. Concurrent medical treatment may take place during the low vision intervention because many conditions may be progressive in nature (including macular degeneration, diabetic retinopathy, or glaucoma).

A detailed case history is the first step in low vision rehabilitation. A common part of present routine medical care is to have the patient complete a preexamination written survey that includes a medical history and a systems analysis (e.g., heart, lungs, kidneys, genitourinary, neurological). A similar survey, which includes functional problems, is helpful before a low vision assessment, but it may be difficult for the patient with low vision to fill out, because people with impaired vision generally have difficulty filling out forms. In these cases, another option is to obtain the intake information over the telephone, before the evaluation. The optometrist or ophthalmologist can then review any problem areas and cover in detail the eye history as well as the medical history.

It is during the telephone intake, or when the clinician reviews the history, that problems other than vision may be manifested. It is normal for people with vision loss to experience symptoms of anger, denial, or depression. Often, success in the vision rehabilitation process depends on the progress made in coming to terms with the vision loss.

The case history comprises patient observation; ocular history; general medical history; living situation; and task analysis of traveling, distance viewing, ADLs, near tasks, lighting, and work- or school-related tasks. Patient objectives are established during the history. The ultimate goal of the evaluation, however, is to provide *prescriptive* optical, electronic, or other adaptive devices along with rehabilitative services, such as orientation and mobility, training in ADLs, or social services intervention when indicated. A prescriptive device can be a spectacle correction, such as distance, near, bifocal, or trifocal lenses. Prescriptive devices also can be hand or stand magnifiers, telescopic systems, absorptive lenses, or electronic magnification systems.

The appropriate strength of a prescriptive device is determined from the low vision evaluation. A loss of ability to use a prescriptive device that previously worked may indicate a serious change in the visual status owing to an active disease process (e.g., hemorrhage, retinal detachment, or increase in the intraocular pressure). These conditions warrant immediate attention.

In infants and children, the low vision history will include not only questions to the parents about the child's visual behavior but also questions about the child's overall development. Because physical, cognitive, and social development are all influenced by vision, a vision problem should be identified early so that, if necessary, other types of intervention can be instituted to assist the child as he or she grows.

The clinician should note any medications, either ocular or systemic, that may affect the functional vision of the patient with low vision. Some of the more common medications include

- Antihistamines,
- Antidepressants,
- Carbonic anhydrase inhibitors,
- Corticosteroids,
- Mydriatic agents,
- Nonsteroidal anti-inflammatory drugs,
- Anti-infective agents, and
- Glaucoma agents.

Medications may affect the visual system as well as the patient's psychological status. Some of the areas that may be affected (Oliver, 1996) are

- Color perception,
- Contrast sensitivity,
- Depth of focus,
- Depth of field,
- Extraocular muscle function (eye movements),
- Lacrimation (tearing or dry eyes),
- Lighting needs,
- Magnification requirement,
- Ocular surface integrity,
- Patient's psychological status,
- Perceived brightness,
- Pupil size,
- Rate of blinking,
- Tear film quality,
- Visual acuity measurement, and
- Visual field.

Oliver (1996) noted that the low vision evaluation should be performed before the instillation of any medications into the patient's eyes to eliminate the risk of adverse reactions that can affect the patient's visual performance. Oliver also noted that all patients using topical steroids need to be closely monitored for the development of elevated intraocular pressure, cataracts, or other complications that could have a detrimental effect on ocular health or efficient visual performance. Problems such as a loss in contrast sensitivity (which is discussed later in this chapter) and a decrease in visual acuity can result.

The history will provide information on the major areas of difficulty, and at the conclusion of the evaluation, recommendations will be made for the appropriate low vision devices or additional services warranted.

Visual Acuity

Visual acuity is a measure of the smallest target an eye can recognize or detect at a specific distance. Visual acuity measurement follows the case history. For a patient with low vision, it is important to determine an *accurate* visual acuity and *not* to use other notations, such as counts fingers or hand motion. These terms do little to describe the visual function.

To enable the accurate measurement of a functional visual acuity, specialized charts are used in the low vision evaluation. These charts take the place of the projector chart found in a typical examination room.

Distance visual acuity measures generally use single letters calibrated according to the distance at which the letters subtend 5 minutes of arc (5′) and each component of the letter subtends 1 minute of arc (1′). (*Note.* 5 minutes of arc is equal to 1/12th of 1°.) The Snellen fraction is given by the test distance in the numerator and standard distance of the smallest letter correctly identified in the denominator.

As noted earlier, the chart generally used in the primary eye examination room is a chart that is projected onto the wall. This chart is often not the best way to measure low levels of visual acuity and therefore does not permit the most accurate measurement of acuities worse than 20/100.

A variety of other charts are preferred for use in the low vision examination. One in frequent use today is known as the *ETDRS chart,* which comes from *Early Treatment of Diabetic Retinopathy Study* (see Figure 2.1). (This is also the standard eye chart used in research for all studies conducted by the National Eye Institute.) The chart's specific properties are
- An equal number of letters (5) on each line,
- A logarithmic progression from line to line,
- An equal level of difficulty on each line (in terms of ability to recognize the letters), and
- An equal spacing between the letters and the lines.

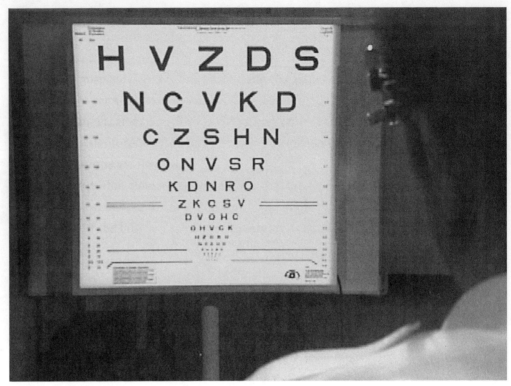

Figure 2.1. ETDRS chart.
From *The Lighthouse Low Vision Examination Techniques,* "Function Tests." Copyright © 1996,
Lighthouse International. Reprinted with permission.

These properties lead to an equal crowding effect at every acuity level, which makes the acuity task the same at all levels of acuity. (*Crowding* occurs when a target is surrounded by other objects, making the object of regard more difficult to see.)

With the ETDRS chart, visual acuity can be accurately measured from as low as 20/800 to as high as 20/20. However, notation of low vision acuity (both distance and near) with the ETDRS chart is done in metric (M) units.

Acuity in metric notation is done the same way as traditional Snellen acuity (which is in foot notation). For example, if the testing is at 2 m, then the numerator of the fraction is 2. If the visual acuity is measured at 4 m, then the numerator is 4. The denominator, as noted previously, would be the size of the smallest letter read at the test distance.

Therefore, if the testing were done at 2 m, and the smallest letter read was the top line of the ETDRS chart, then that person's visual acuity would be 2/40. Conversion to Snellen acuity is easily accomplished. In this example, adding a 0 to the digits of the numerator and denominator would give an equivalent Snellen acuity of 20/400. If the smallest line read were the 20M-size letter at 2 m, then the acuity would be 2/20 (equivalent to 20/200).

Another low vision chart in common usage is the *Designs for Vision* or *Feinbloom number chart* (Figure 2.2), which has numbers as large as 700 ft, allowing the doctor to measure visual acuities that are even lower than with the ETDRS chart. As an illustration,

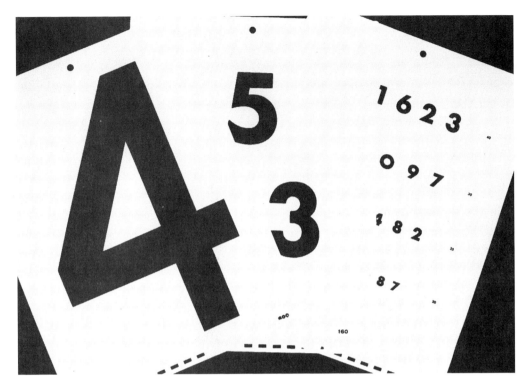

Figure 2.2. Designs for vision number chart.
Photo courtesy of Richard Feinbloom, president, Designs for Vision, Ronkonkoma, NY. Reprinted with permission.

if the largest number read is the 700-ft number, and the patient can see it only at 1 ft away, then the visual acuity is 1/700, which is equivalent to 20/14,000. It is important to note that the testing distance and the letters used to take the acuity must be measured in the same units (i.e., both in meters or both in feet; one cannot mix the two units in a single fraction).

When evaluating acuity with these larger targets (whether by ETDRS, Designs for Vision, or some other acuity chart), people may be encouraged to use the part of their vision that allows them to see more clearly. Patients with loss of central vision may need to intentionally look off to the side to make out the letters on the chart, a technique known as *eccentric viewing*. People with inherited vision loss frequently use these off-center points instinctively, whereas those with an acquired vision loss may need training or prisms to help them find the point that allows optimal visual performance.

Near visual acuity is taken at the habitual reading distance (where the patient normally reads). For instance, if the patient routinely holds the reading material 3 in. from the nose, the low vision doctor will begin taking near acuities at this distance. Near acuities will be taken at specific distances later in the examination to help determine how much magnification the patient will need for various near tasks. The importance of lighting control may be initially addressed during this phase of the testing, as illumination can be critical to the patient's success with low vision devices.

Visual acuity also can be measured (or at least estimated) in infants and young children with low vision by using specialized testing procedures. The procedures used will depend on the child's age and responsiveness. One such test is *preferential looking,* in which grating patterns (stripes) are presented in front of the child to one side, with no pattern on the other side. Sometimes other targets are used. The basis of the test is that if the child can see the pattern, he or she will prefer to look in that direction. If the child reacts positively to the cards with the smaller stripes, this suggests better visual acuity. The person performing the test must be trained to perform it properly and to interpret the child's responses. Other tests that use symbols (see, for example, Figure 2.3), instead of letters or numbers, can be used with more responsive children to more accurately estimate visual acuity.

Refraction

Refraction is the procedure used to determine which lenses are needed to accurately focus light from distant objects on the retina. In simpler terms, it is the way the doctor determines whether the patient is farsighted or nearsighted or has astigmatism (which can cause blurry vision at all distances).

A careful refraction is essential before any determination of the appropriate lens system. Significant changes in the refraction may be caused by cataract formation or other ocular changes. Specialized techniques are often used in the low vision examination in the determination of the refractive error, because these patients may be viewing eccentrically, have media interference from the cornea or the lens, or have high uncorrected refractive error.

In low vision, a trial frame often is used for the refraction instead of the standard *phoropter,* which is the instrument with many lenses used in the primary care evaluation. The subjective evaluation (in which the doctor gives the patient a variety of lens choices to more accurately determine the appropriate lens prescription) may result in a prescription that is significantly different from the entering prescription. This difference may be due to physiologic changes in the eye or to the fact that the patient has not undergone an accurate refraction.

When a patient is too young to respond to lens choices, or is noncommunicative for some other reason (as occurs sometimes after a stroke), a refractive evaluation still can be performed by the optometrist or ophthalmologist using a procedure called *retinoscopy.* By shining a light in the eye and using different lenses, the doctor can frequently get a very accurate, objective determination of the refractive error.

Predicting the Magnification

Following the refraction, the clinician will use specialized charts to determine the appropriate magnification for achieving the patient's objectives. These objectives may include

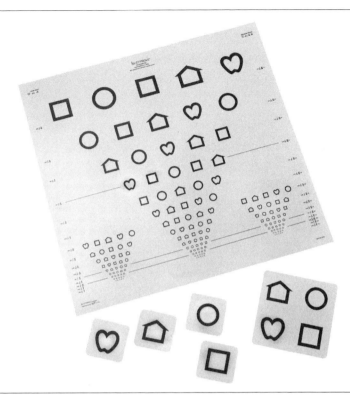

Figure 2.3. Lea symbols.
Photo courtesy of Chris Greening, chief executive officer, Good-Lite®, Streamwood, IL. Reprinted with permission.

everyday tasks like reading the daily newspaper, looking at prices or labels, reading the mail, or even loading a syringe (if the patient has diabetes).

As noted earlier, low vision clinicians use M notation to record near visual acuity. A 1M letter is a letter subtending 5 minutes of arc when held at a distance of 1 m. A 1M letter, which is generally considered to be the size of newspaper print, is comparable to a 20/50 Snellen letter, or 9-point type when it is viewed at 16 in. (40 cm). A 2M letter is twice the size of a 1M letter.

Other Tests of Visual Function

Amsler Grid and Contrast Sensitivity

The *Amsler grid* (see Figure 2.4) and *contrast sensitivity evaluation* (see Figure 2.5) follow the refraction. The Amsler grid is a standard diagnostic test used to help identify early macular changes. However, the Amsler grid has a different function in the low vision evaluation than the primary care examination. It is used as a prognostic indicator of a patient's success with low vision devices.

The grid, when viewed at 33 cm (13 in.), reflects the integrity of the central 20° of vision. It is an important test that demonstrates the position and density of *scotomas* (areas of no vision) and whether the patient should be using the right eye, left eye, or both eyes. Patients who have experienced changes in the macula from hemorrhaging, scarring, edema, or laser treatment may exhibit such scotomas. Damage to other structures in the visual pathway (e.g., the optic nerve) also can lead to scotomas.

Contrast sensitivity testing also is important in determining the patient's visual function. Two methods are used clinically to assess a person's contrast sensitivity: (a) sine wave gratings of different spatial frequencies that decrease in contrast across the chart and (b) letters or symbols of decreasing contrast. The method with gratings is similar to a hearing test in which a person's high, middle, and low hearing frequencies are determined. Using letters of decreasing contrast gives somewhat less-detailed information, but it is still very useful clinically, and the letter–symbol tests are often quicker and easier to administer.

Contrast sensitivity tests can provide valuable information on the effect of lighting for reading as well as determine whether increased magnification is necessary for near visual tasks. Contrast testing also is beneficial in predicting whether an individual may perform better with white letters on a black background (reverse polarity) and can explain some of the difficulties that a person has with ADLs (e.g., seeing the edges of a dinner plate, seeing cracks in the sidewalk).

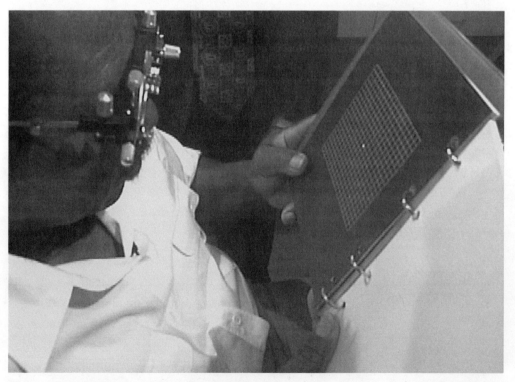

Figure 2.4. A patient being tested with an Amsler grid.
From *The Lighthouse Low Vision Examination Techniques,* "Function Tests." Copyright © 1996, Lighthouse International. Reprinted with permission.

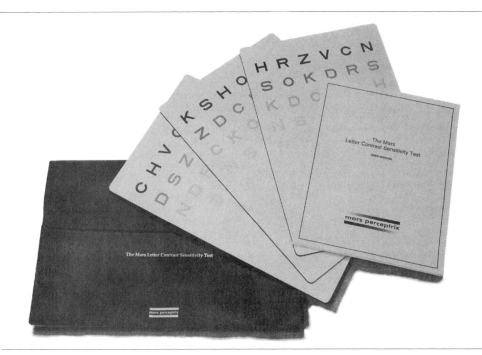

Figure 2.5. The Mars Letter Contrast Sensitivity Test.
Photo courtesy of Aries Arditi, PhD, Chappaqua, NY. Reprinted with permission.

Visual Field Assessment

Visual field analysis provides subjective information on the extent of the loss of peripheral or central visual field (see Figure 2.6). Some of the primary uses of the visual field analysis in the low vision examination are to

- Establish whether an individual is legally blind,
- Determine whether the visual field is large enough so that the person can drive legally,
- Establish a baseline for monitoring future change,
- Serve as an aid in the selection of low vision devices, and
- Identify the need for orientation and mobility training (Nowakowski, 1994).

A variety of techniques are used to determine the extent of a person's visual field loss. The Amsler grid, described earlier, provides information on the central 20° of the visual field. The *tangent screen* is another central field technique that evaluates the central 30° of the visual field, although it is not used frequently anymore. More sophisticated equipment is used to determine the visual field for driving or the progression of a visual field loss. The most commonly used visual field plotters are the *automated visual field units* and the *Goldmann perimeter* (but the latter are much less available than in the past).

Bass and Sherman (1996) stated that automated perimetry has paved the way for more standardized and accurate visual field testing in all types of patients, including those with low vision. They also pointed out that, although automated perimetry makes it relatively easy to perform visual field testing, the interpretation still lies with the practitioner.

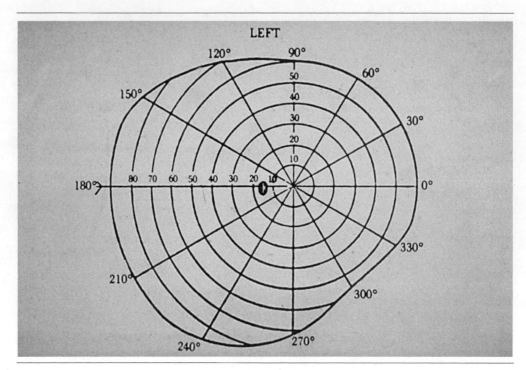

Figure 2.6. Diagrammatic representation of the extent of the normal visual field in the left eye.

A visual field screening in infants and young children is possible. Evaluation may involve the use of colored objects or lights. Although the test in young children is often less accurate and more qualitative than quantitative, it is still possible to get a sense of whether a child has a significant visual field loss.

Color Vision Testing

Fischer (1996) noted two reasons for considering color vision testing in the patient with low vision:

1. *Diagnosis.* Color test results, in conjunction with other examination findings, can sometimes be an invaluable part of a diagnostic profile, where the etiology of a patient's vision loss is uncertain. For example, hereditary (congenital) defects are usually found in males, are red–green in nature, and show predictable and repeatable results, whereas acquired color deficiencies may be found in males or females, are blue–yellow or red–green, are unpredictable, and often are not repeatable.
2. *Function.* Some patients may depend on color vision for certain tasks in their daily lives.

Most commercially available color vision tests were designed to detect and classify hereditary color vision deficiencies; as such, they may have limited value for a patient with low vision. One of the more commonly used and beneficial color vision tests in the assessment of the patient with low vision is the *Farnsworth Panel D-15 test*, in which the patient is asked to put colored caps in a specific order. Although many people with low vision can perform the regular D-15 test, versions of the D-15 test that have larger stimuli have been developed (e.g., Hyvarinen, (1995). A similar but more-extensive and time-consuming test of color perception is the *Farnsworth–Munsell 100-Hue test,* also a color-ordering task.

Individuals may experience color vision loss when a specific part of the visual system is affected. For example, people with macular degeneration, glaucoma, and diabetic retinopathy may demonstrate a blue–yellow defect, whereas those with optic nerve disease may reveal a red–green defect. Pharmaceutical agents also may cause a change on the color vision tests. For example, people on certain medications for cardiovascular problems may demonstrate either a blue–yellow or a red–green defect and may report yellow vision.

Ocular Health Assessment

An ocular health assessment is done to determine the type and extent of disease present in the eyes and associated structures. A gross assessment is often performed early in the low vision evaluation (after visual acuities) to identify any obvious abnormalities that might affect the functional portions of the examination. This external evaluation will include the pupillary reactions; ocular motility; evaluation of strabismus; the presence of nystagmus; and the appearance of the lids, cornea, and iris. More detailed testing, including biomicroscopy and ophthalmoscopy (described earlier), is generally performed at the very end of the low vision evaluation to thoroughly assess all ocular structures.

Selecting the Appropriate Low Vision Device

Once the history, refraction, and functional assessment are complete, the clinician takes all the information and uses it to test and select the appropriate optical or adaptive device that will allow the patient to achieve his or her objectives. First, the doctor must determine whether a standard distance correction, bifocals, or reading glasses should be prescribed. This is followed by an assessment of the patient's performance with various low vision devices and the ultimate selection of the appropriate low vision device(s) to help the patient.

Low vision devices are grouped into the following categories:
- High plus spectacle lenses,
- Hand magnifiers,
- Stand magnifiers,
- Telescopes,
- Absorptive lenses,
- Field "expanders,"
- Electronic magnification systems, and
- Adaptive (nonoptical) devices.

Because low vision optical devices frequently require training to use them successfully, it is common to let patients have a trial period with the device(s) at home before making a final decision on the device to be prescribed. The doctor and patient, along with the low vision instructor, will work together to arrive at the most appropriate devices to address the patient's different needs.

Basic Optics

Lenses are designated in plus and minus *power* (e.g., +5.00, −5.00). Plus (+) lenses are prescribed over the distance refraction to focus the person on near objects. The lenses primarily used in low vision remediation are strong plus (+) lenses.

The standard unit of measurement to describe the power of a lens, whether it is prescribed for distance vision or near vision, is the *diopter*. One diopter of lens power will focus parallel light 1 m away. The larger the number of diopters, the stronger the lens. For example, a +5.00 diopter lens is twice as strong as a +2.50 diopter lens, and a +10.00 lens is twice as strong as a +5.00 lens. Exceptionally strong lenses may be used in low vision remediation (e.g., +10.00 diopters to +80.00 diopters).

Another concept is the *focal length* of the lens: The stronger the lens, the shorter the focal length and the closer the reading material must be held to get it in focus. An easy way to visualize the focal length of a plus lens is to think of a leaf being burned by a magnifier. The stronger the magnifier, the closer it has to be held to the leaf.

The following are some illustrations of the focal length of lenses:

* A +2.50 diopter lens will focus at 40 cm (16 in.) to burn the leaf.
* A +5.00 diopter lens will focus at 20 cm (8 in.).
* A +10.00 diopter lens will focus at 10 cm (4 in.).
* A +20.00 diopter lens will focus at 5 cm (2 in.).
* A +40.00 diopter lens will focus at 2.5 cm (1 in.).

Some general rules can be applied when working with patients with low vision:

* The poorer the vision, the stronger the lens prescribed.
* The stronger the lens, the closer to the page one has to work.
* The stronger the lens, the more critical the lighting will be while reading.
* The stronger the lens, the smaller the area that one can see while reading (i.e., an individual with normal vision can scan a line, whereas a person with a severe visual impairment might be able to read only a few letters at one time).
* Reading becomes progressively more difficult as the strength of the lens increases.

High Plus Spectacles, Hand Magnifiers, and Stand Magnifiers

The plus lens is prescribed in three forms that have equivalent power (strength). Specifically, the lens can be put into a pair of glasses known as a *high plus* or *microscopic spectacle*; it can be placed into a more traditional hand magnifier; or it can be put in a rigid housing, known as a *stand magnifier*, which is placed onto the reading material.

High plus or microscopic spectacles are the most commonly prescribed low vision devices for close work. They offer the benefit of looking like normal glasses, and they allow the hands to be free for holding reading material or other objects. Depending on the findings of the function tests, they may be prescribed for binocular (two-eyes) or monocular (one-eye) use. In general, binocular corrections are given to people with vision better than 20/200. The most frequently prescribed binocular reading lenses used in low vision are the prism half-eye glasses (see Figure 2.7), which are generally prescribed up to +12.00 diopters.

High plus spectacles (see Figure 2.8) also may be prescribed monocularly, especially when vision is significantly decreased. The most commonly prescribed microscopic lens is known as the *aspheric lens* (a lens with special curves to correct for aberrations in its periphery). Up to 12x magnification (+48 diopters) is prescribed.

In addition to the aspheric lens, more sophisticated systems known as the *doublet lenses* (lenses composed of two plus lenses separated by an air space) are used. Doublet lenses (shown in Figure 2.8) have better optics and a wider usable field for reading. A common doublet lens that is prescribed is the Clear Image lens, manufactured by Designs for Vision.

Hand magnifiers are used for common short-term activities, such as looking at prices, labels, recipes, oven dials, bills, or telephone numbers. They come in powers ranging from 1.5x to 20x magnification (6–80 diopters).

A variety of hand magnifiers are available. They range from inexpensive spherical magnifiers that generally have poor optics to sophisticated aspheric and multiple lens systems with superior optics. Prescription of the hand magnifier is again dependent on the patient's needs and the findings from the functional evaluative tests.

Stand magnifiers are hand-held devices but, unlike hand magnifiers, which require focusing by the user, stand magnifiers sit directly on the reading material, eliminating the need for the patient to find the focal distance. They can be very useful for patients who have hand tremors and thus cannot hold a hand magnifier or reading material steady. The optics of stand magnifiers are more complex than some of the other low vision devices, and expertise is required in selecting the appropriate power magnifier and the appropriate prescription lenses to be used in conjunction with the magnifier.

Telescopes

Patients with low vision frequently need assistance in seeing things more clearly at a distance. Unfortunately, these patients do not always receive sufficient improvement in a distance vision from standard distance glasses, because it is not possible to magnify with standard spectacles. The only way that distant objects can be magnified is with a telescopic system.

Telescopes come in a variety of styles and powers. Many patients with low vision will use hand-held telescopes for spotting tasks involved with mobility (e.g., reading street

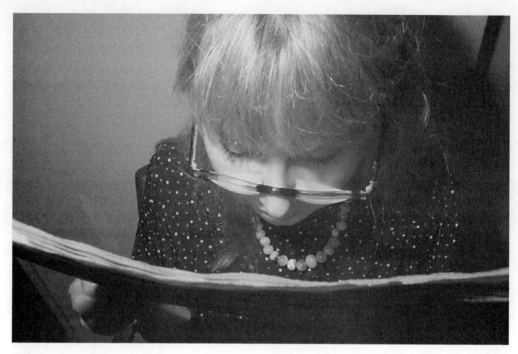

Figure 2.7. Half-eye prism glasses.
Copyright © 1996, Lighthouse International. Reprinted with permission.

signs, seeing traffic lights and "Walk" and "Don't Walk" signals). Spectacle-mounted telescopes often are used for tasks in which the person needs to use the telescope for extended periods or for tasks in which the hands need to be free, such as driving, seeing at the theater, seeing the blackboard in school, and reading music. As with other low vision devices, the patient often needs training to use a telescope successfully.

Absorptive Lenses

Many patients with low vision are photophobic, or experience disability caused by various lighting conditions. This light sensitivity can be the result of several eye conditions, such as a corneal dystrophy, cataract, aniridia (absence of the iris), irregular pupil, albinism, or achromatopsia. Light sensitivity also can be caused by medication or occur after extensive laser treatment to the retina.

Typical questions asked on a case history include inquiries about glare and light sensitivity. It is usual to ask whether the sun is tolerated, whether a cloudy day or a sunny day is more comfortable for the patient, whether sunglasses are worn and if they are effective, and whether seeing in dim light is a problem.

Absorptive lenses are filters that can be worn both indoors and outdoors to reduce the glare and increase contrast. Some of these lenses are specially made to transmit only certain wavelengths of light, thus eliminating glare without making things too dark. They may come as wraparounds or clip-ons and can be polarizing lenses as well. Two of these

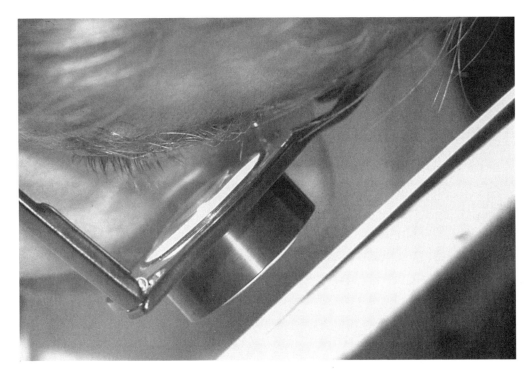

Figure 2.8. High plus microscopic lens.
Copyright © 1996, Lighthouse International. Reprinted with permission.

more specialized absorptive lenses are those from NoIR Medical Technologies and photochromic prescriptive lenses made by Corning.

Electronic Magnification Systems

Perhaps the most significant and rapid advancements have been in the area of electronic magnification systems. Electronic systems may work better for individuals who have more reduced levels of visual function (e.g., acuity less than 20/400, large scotomas requiring eccentric viewing, very reduced contrast sensitivity, or some combination of these).

Traditional in-line closed-circuit television systems have been around for decades. Desktop systems consist of a camera (stationary mounted) that projects an image onto a television monitor. Closed-circuit televisions offer certain advantages over and above optical low vision devices.

- High amounts of magnification are possible; depending on the system, viewing distance, and monitor, magnification can be achieved to greater than 50x. Optical systems are generally available to 20x but are often difficult to use above 5x.
- Polarity can be reversed. Images can be projected onto the screen that are white on black or black on white; this can be especially important to a patient with poor contrast.

- Brightness, contrast, and color presentation can be controlled.
- Newer closed-circuit television systems are available that have many other features, including autofocus technology and speech recognition.

More recently, several developments have made electronic magnification more affordable, and others have made it more portable. These include

- Hand-held cameras that interface with a regular television set, a flat panel display, or head-mounted display;
- Head-mounted systems that have a camera, and small displays in front of each eye, to allow electronic magnification at distance and near;
- Small electronic systems that combine a camera and a flat panel display for use in a library, at school, or when traveling; and
- Miniature LCD magnifiers that can be carried around for spot reading tasks.

It also should be noted that there have been major advances in computer software and hardware since the early 1990s, such that computers have made information much more accessible to a person with a visual impairment. Information on the computer can be more easily accessed through the use of variable screen magnification, speech output, refreshable Braille displays, or combinations of these. Additionally, it can be easier to access typewritten materials by scanning them into the computer and then using screen magnification or a screen reader (speech).

Adaptive (Nonoptical) Devices

Many nonoptical aids can benefit an individual with a visual impairment; these include large-print watches, clocks, and timers; cassette players; television accessories; large-print books and cookbooks; writing supplies; special calculators; measuring tools; money identifiers and wallets; temperature gauges; special telephones; lighting; games; and mobility aids. Among the many health care aids are blood-glucose-monitoring systems and other devices for people with diabetes, voice output thermometers and scales and other voice output devices, and pill dispensers. The low vision doctor or instructor will recommend these types of assistive devices, in addition to the prescriptive optical devices, to try to address the patient's needs.

Outcomes of the Low Vision Examination

On the basis of all the testing performed, the doctor will work with the patient to come up with appropriate solutions to address the different problems. These may include

- Prescription of glasses;
- Prescription of low vision devices;
- Referrals for other vision rehabilitation services to address problems related to ADLs, orientation, and mobility;
- A referral for training related to vocational or educational concerns; and
- A referral for counseling when the person or family is having difficulty coping with the loss of vision.

Additionally, as noted earlier, supplemental tests (e.g., VEP, ERG) can be ordered in cases in which additional diagnostic information is required to help manage the patient, and patients also will be referred back to their primary eye care provider if changes in their eye condition are present.

Finally, an important component is that the doctor will provide the patient with information about the patient's disease and how it affects his or her function, as well as ways to address the problems resulting from the functional loss. The ultimate goal of low vision rehabilitation is to allow the patient to improve function and regain independence.

References

Arditi, A., & Rosenthal, B. P. (1996, July). *Developing an objective definition of visual impairment.* Paper presented at Vision 96, the International Conference on Low Vision, Madrid, Spain.

Bass, S. J., & Sherman, J. (1991). Ophthalmic ultrasonography. In J. B. Eskridge, J. F. Amos, & J. D. Bartlett (Eds.), *Clinical procedures in optometry* (pp. 530–549). Philadelphia: Lippincott.

Bass, S. J., & Sherman, J. (1996). Visual field testing in the low vision patient. In B. P. Rosenthal & R. G. Cole (Eds.), *Functional assessment of low vision* (pp. 89–104). St. Louis, MO: Mosby.

Colenbrander, A. (1976). Low vision: Definition and classification. In E. E. Faye (Ed.), *Clinical low vision* (pp. 3–6). Boston: Little, Brown.

Dana, M. R., Tielsch, J. M., Enger, C., Joyce, E., Santoli, J. M., & Taylor, H. R. (1990). Visual impairment in a rural Appalachian community. *Journal of the American Medical Association, 264,* 2400–2405.

Faye, E. E. (1984). *Clinical low vision.* Boston: Little, Brown.

Fingeret, M., Casser, L., & Woodcome, H. T. (1990). *Atlas of primary eyecare procedures.* Norwalk, CT: Appleton & Lange.

Fischer, M. L. (1996). Clinical implications of color vision deficiencies. In B. P. Rosenthal & R. G. Cole (Eds.), *Functional assessment of low vision* (pp. 105–128). St. Louis, MO: Mosby.

Hyvarinen, L. (1995). Considerations in evaluation and treatment of the child with low vision. *American Journal of Occupational Therapy, 49,* 896.

Johnston, A. W. (1991). Making sense of the M, N, and logMAR systems of specifying visual acuity. In B. P. Rosenthal & R. G. Cole (Eds.), *Problems in optometry: A structured approach to low vision care* (Vol. 3, No. 3, pp. 394–407). Philadelphia: Lippincott.

Kahn, H. A., Leibowitz. H. M., Ganley, J. P., Kini, M. M., Colton, T., Nickerson, R. S., et al. (1977). The Framingham Eye Study: Vol. 1. Outline and major prevalence findings. *American Journal of Epidemiology, 106,* 17–32.

Klein, R., Klein, B. E. K., Linton, K. L. P., & De Mets, D. L. (1991). The Beaver Dam Eye Study: Visual acuity. *Ophthalmology, 98,* 1310–1315.

Mehr, E., & Freid, A. (1975). *Low vision care.* Chicago: Professional Press.

New York Lighthouse (now Lighthouse International). (1974). *Low vision examination* [Low vision continuing education curriculum]. New York: Author.

Nowakowski, R. (1994). *Primary low vision care.* Norwalk, CT: Appleton & Lange.

Oliver, G. E. (1996). Pharmaceutical effects on the management of the low vision patient. In R. G. Cole & B. P. Rosenthal (Eds.), *Remediation and management of the low vision patient* (pp. 123–138). St. Louis, MO: Mosby.

Oshinskie, L. J. (1991). Radiology. In J. B. Eskridge, J. F. Amos, & J. D. Bartlett (Eds.), *Clinical procedures in optometry* (pp. 580–595). Philadelphia: Lippincott.

Sherman, J., & Bass, S. J. (1984). Diagnostic procedures in low vision case management. In E. E. Faye (Ed.), *Clinical low vision* (pp. 226–227). Boston: Little, Brown.

Sherman, J., & Bass, S. J. (1996). Electrodiagnosis in evaluation and managing the low vision patient. In B. P. Rosenthal & R. G. Cole (Eds.), *Functional assessment of low vision* (pp. 140, 148–157). St. Louis, MO: Mosby.

Sherman, J., & Sutija, V. G. (1991). Visual-evoked potentials. In J. B. Eskridge, J. F. Amos, & J. D. Bartlett (Eds.), *Clinical procedures in optometry* (pp. 514–529). Philadelphia: Lippincott.

Tielsch, J. M., Sommer, A., Witt, K., Katz, J., & Royall, R. M. (1990). Blindness and visual impairment in an American urban population: The Baltimore Eye Study. *Archives of Ophthalmology, 108,* 286–290.

U.S. Bureau of the Census. (1989). *Population profile of the United States: 1989* (Current Population Reports, Series P-23, No. 159). Washington, DC: U.S. Government Printing Office.

Additional Reading

Bailey, I. L. (1988). Measurement of visual acuity—Towards standardization. In *Vision Science Symposium* (pp. 215–230). Bloomington: Indiana University Press.

Colenbrander, A. (1977). Dimensions of visual performance. *Transactions of the American Academy of Ophthalmology and Otolaryngology, 83,* 322.

Colenbrander, A., & Fletcher, D. C. (1995). Basic concepts and terms for low vision rehabilitation. *American Journal of Occupational Therapy, 49,* 865–869.

Rosenthal, B. P., & Cole, R. G. (1993). Visual impairments. In M. G. Eisenberg, R. L. Glueckauf, & H. Zaretsky (Eds.), *Medical aspects of disability* (pp. 391–403). New York: Springer.

Functional Aspects of the
Eye Diagnosis in Older Adults

Eleanor E. Faye, MD, FACS

Older adults typically have a variety of deficits, both physical and cognitive. They may be taking several medications, and side effects may be a significant factor in their general adaptation to aging. One of the most difficult and important functions that must be factored in when starting a rehabilitation program of any type is the visual status of the person. Self-reporting of vision problems is notoriously inaccurate: A person who says "I don't see very well" may be expressing only a need for a new prescription of glasses for distance vision or perhaps stronger reading glasses, but in addition to these normal aging changes he or she also may have the early stages of cataracts, glaucoma, or macular degeneration.

Any patient who is experiencing vision changes is at a disadvantage if the therapist who is formulating a rehabilitation plan does not know the extent of the patient's visual abilities and does not have access to the results of a complete eye examination. Depending on the diagnosis, the rehabilitation professional who understands the implications of the person's eye problem can incorporate special techniques into the rehabilitation plan, if necessary, or help the patient adapt to low vision devices that may enhance the rehabilitation process. For example, a stroke patient who is being taught to use a microwave oven but cannot see the settings is not being well served when there exist devices that can improve his or her near vision.

Many eye complaints prove to be easily solved, but an eye symptom cannot be ignored and blamed on age until it is proven to be innocuous. The basic problem is that many aging adults have changes in their sight that are the result of normal aging, but the same symptoms also could be a warning of eye pathology. Regardless of the complaint, and whether the solution is eyeglasses, surgery, or medications, everyone needs a baseline evaluation.

Symptoms and their functional implications must be evaluated by eye care professionals, ophthalmologists, or optometrists. If a person has irreversible vision loss, this *low vision patient* should be referred to a vision rehabilitation eye care professional for evaluation and prescription of remedial devices. The need for a subsequent instruction program involves a knowledgeable therapist who is trained in vision rehabilitation. The functional evaluation should answer the following questions:

- What is the functional extent of the eye diseases?
- How does the patient's attitude affect prognosis for successful rehabilitation?
- What environmental changes are needed (e.g., lighting, contrast, print size)?
- Must tasks be modified? If so, how?
- What optical devices are useful, and will the patient be able to learn to use them to accomplish objectives?
- How does the person's physical condition (e.g., other diagnoses with implications for use of limbs, balance, motivation) affect the use of optical devices?
- What are the patient's goals, and are they realistic?

The first section of this chapter will describe normal aging changes and typical symptoms associated with these changes. The second section will cover symptoms and functional characteristics for three groups of eye diseases. The symptoms unique to each group and suggested ways the rehabilitation process must be tailored to moderate these different symptoms will be described. The next section will discuss the low vision evaluation, emphasizing the tests that are not included in a standard eye examination. The final section describes devices that are appropriate for each group and that apply to the remediation of the patient's symptoms.

Visual Changes Associated With Normal Aging

Is there such a thing as "normal" aging of the eye? Can function decrease without ocular disease? The answers are not clear cut, because many changes in the eye do not initially affect visual activity or acuity. As everyday activities for an aging person decrease, visual demands also decrease, so that the person is unaware of a visual malfunction (Marmor, 1995). In addition, aging does not affect all people or all systems uniformly or equally. Therefore, it is imperative to differentiate between changes due to aging versus changes due to outright pathology.

Results from the Framingham Study (Liebowitz et al., 1980) dispel the myth that all aging persons can expect to have an eye disease eventually. Of the most common conditions—cataract, macular degeneration, glaucoma, and diabetic retinopathy—only 19% of adults between ages 65 and 74 years have at least one disease. After age 75, the number increases to 50% as the prevalence of age-related cataract and macular degeneration increases. But this means that a significant number of older adults can remain free of functional deficits well into their 80s. The aging baby boomers may change the demographics of aging because of their more rigorous control of cholesterol, blood pressure, and a healthier diet, although this may be offset by the increasing obesity statistics.

Aging of the Lens, Cornea, and Vitreous

Optical media changes associated with normal aging occur in the lens, cornea, and vitreous. As these clear structures age, they develop microscopic changes in the protein molecules (Faye, 2000). Minute particles absorb light and scatter short-wave light rays (blue or ultraviolet; Wolf, 1960). These microscopic changes reduce the quantity of light reaching the retina and, more significantly, cause glare from light sources, such as headlights, street lamps, bright lights, and windows. When working with older adults, it is important to note the level of illumination and type of lamp that provide the most comfort, the best illumination without glare, as well as good contrast. For example, a person may require more light for reading but complain of glare when fluorescent or halogen lights reflect from the page of a magazine printed on shiny paper (Hemenger, 1984). Incandescent light generally provides less fatigue and more comfort than high-intensity lamps, and the person should be instructed to position the light source in front of the face rather than from either side behind the head.

Another structural change in older people may be a small pupil due to loss of sphincter muscle tone of the iris or a pupil that has become small and atrophic because of taking glaucoma medication (pilocarpine) for many years. When the pupil can no longer dilate in response to low-light conditions, a delay in dark and light adaptation occurs. This delay becomes significant with hallway lighting; orientation on entering an unfamiliar building or room; or safe traveling in bad weather, driving, or traveling at night.

Presbyopia

So-called *middle-aged sight*, or *presbyopia* ("old eye"), is well known to people in their mid- to late 40s, unless they are myopic and can read without their distance glasses. In youth, the lens of the eye responds promptly to a near object by contraction of the muscle of accommodation in the eye, which allows the lens to become more convex (i.e., stronger) to accommodate for the greater power needed for near work. Most near work involves print, computer images, and drawings. As the lens becomes more rigid with age, it becomes less and less elastic so that, even if the muscle contracts, it can no longer become convex enough for the near task. This deficiency can be simply remedied by the prescription of reading glasses in whatever form best suits the person's needs: single reading lenses, half-eye frames, bifocals, trifocals, and progressive lenses. The spectacle lenses basically provide new convex lenses strong enough to focus the eye for reading and intermediate distance. Some people require distance glasses as well, when the eyes cannot even accommodate for that range without help (Hofstetter, 1965).

Visual Acuity

As the eye ages, it may require a prescription lens to see clearly not only for near range but also for distance and the intermediate (arm's-length) range as well. As a rule, eyes become more farsighted (hyperopic) with age, resulting in the inability to focus clearly for any distance. A myopic (nearsighted) person tends to have worn glasses for distance for many years yet becomes more farsighted (less myopic) with age. This requires a change of reading habits, such as removing distance glasses to read, or resorting to using a separate pair of reading glasses. The implication of this tendency to become farsighted is that refraction should be repeated at approximately 2-year intervals to be sure that the prescription is up to date and that the person is not blaming incorrect glasses on the notion that "Well, I guess I'm just getting old" (Owsley & Sloan, 1980).

Before starting with a rehabilitation program of any kind, it is important for the therapist to know which glasses the patient uses for which activity and whether the prescription is current, the glasses are clean and scratch free, and the frame fits. Consider a situation in which a patient is reported to have 20/20 vision yet does not seem to see details. What does that signify? It is important when evaluating a person's performance to realize that a standard acuity test, which is based on high-contrast letters, bears so little resemblance to the real world that a person's self-reported history is more significant than an acuity measure. Performance either can be better than the acuity might suggest or, in some instances, worse—and the therapist should know the reason. Is the cause age, or an eye disease? The essential point is to insist that people have complete eye examinations to explain complaints rather than blame old age for poor performance.

Contrast

Aging reduces older adults' ability to discern objects against a background of a similar or related color, for example, a cut out edge of a curb, gray concrete steps without a clearly marked edge, stairs with carpeting that has a confusing pattern. Several factors are involved in the waning of contrast perception, such as structural changes in the cornea or lens as well as a diminished sensitivity of retinal receptors. Contrast is further reduced in the presence of cataracts, corneal disease, glaucoma, and retinal pathology (Owsley, Sekuler, & Siemsen, 1983).

When working with older adults—whether the activity is selecting the color of thread and fabric, arranging a place setting, serving food on a plate of contrasting color, reading low-contrast newspaper print, watching television, or working with a computer—contrast must always be a prime consideration. Opposites such as black and white offer the best contrast, but contrasting a dark against a light color, such as blue against white and yellow against violet, is more effective than, say, orange against red, which are too close to each other in the color spectrum to provide enough contrast (Arditi, 2002).

Color Vision

Color vision changes with age only if there is an alteration in the cornea or lens tissue. The aging cornea may not transmit light as efficiently, and if the lens becomes pale yellow, which is a typical aging change, colors in the blue–yellow range may be affected. Light blue may be seen as aqua; yellow objects may appear white; navy blue may be seen as black. An older person may want to label clothes that are easily mismatched. Another potentially serious problem is identifying pills and medications by color rather than by shape, size, or a clearly marked label. A yellow pill may appear white or beige. A blue pill may appear to be light green, and a red pill may appear to be brown.

Visual Field

With age comes a gradual inattention to objects in the peripheral field of view. Not only does sensitivity of the retina diminish with age, but older people also experience a reduction in awareness of activities in the periphery. Because of this unawareness or delayed recognition of movement in the outer field of view, many older people are involved in automobile crashes at intersections (Ball, Owsley, & Beard, 1989). Older people have to be cautioned to be especially alert to hazards and moving objects while walking and driving. Slower reaction time is often part of the inattention.

No Longer Normal Aging, But Low Vision

At some point in an older person's life the aging process may progress to actual pathology. Symptoms cease being simply a nuisance and begin interfering with activities that were once routine. If an examination reveals pathology that cannot be corrected either medically or surgically, or with conventional eyeglass correction, the resulting decrease in visual function is called *low vision*, and its management is called *vision rehabilitation*.

Common Eye Diseases and Visual Function

Before the low vision evaluation, function tests and the prescription of devices to aid in rehabilitation are discussed, eye pathology must be explained in terms of the effect that it has on function tests; the implication of the low vision evaluation, and the tests of visual function will make more sense after one first studies the various ways eye diseases can affect visual function. The presence of an eye disease influences not only what the doctor can prescribe but also what the therapist can expect to accomplish in regard to vision rehabilitation. The type and degree of disease even limit the type of device that can be effectively used. The patient's response can only be as good as the level of visual function, regardless of the motivation and enthusiasm on the part of both patient and therapist. The therapist should know what the major and complicating diagnoses are and be able to place the conditions into one or more of the three functional categories.

Three major functional categories exist, and each one has specific symptoms that affect the approach to the design of a rehabilitation plan (Faye, 1996). The three groups include all of the structures of the eye, visual pathways, and visual cortex of the brain. The following description of the three groups includes the structures involved and the visual functions they represent.

1. Group 1, *cloudy optical media,* includes any corneal disease, papillary abnormalities, and all types of cataracts as well as opacities of the vitreous humor (hemorrhage). The optical media (cornea, pupil, lens, and vitreous) are responsible for the focusing of light on the macula as well as screening ultraviolet (short) rays of light.

2. Group 2, *central visual defects,* includes all types of degenerative diseases of the macula, which is the central area of the retina responsible for detail sight, color vision, and adaptation to light. In addition to the dry or wet form of macular degeneration, patients may have macular edema from diabetes mellitus, macular cysts and holes, infections of the macula, and neurological central blind spots from optic nerve disease.

3. Group 3, *peripheral field defects,* includes advanced glaucoma; advanced retinitis pigmentosa (RP); diabetic retinopathy with either peripheral hemorrhages or laser treatment in that area; postsurgical detached retina; stroke; and any other damage to the optic pathways or brain, such as brain tumors. The peripheral retina is responsible for seeing the movement of objects in the periphery (which is important when driving or walking on a crowded street); its cells provide night vision. Its importance in providing spatial orientation cannot be overemphasized. Without peripheral vision, one cannot walk around easily, nor should one drive. The peripheral retina also warns the macula to look directly at a perceived threat and initiate some form of reaction: "Here comes a taxi jumping the red light—get out of the way!" Individuals with peripheral field defects often carry a white mobility cane to alert others to a vision problem.

Every eye condition can be placed into one of these three categories, with the exception of diabetic eye disease, which potentially belongs in any or all of the three categories: a diabetic cataract under Group 1, macular edema under Group 2, and peripheral hemorrhagic or laser retinal damage under Group 3. The object of the three groups is to separate the diseases according to their effect on visual function, which is different for each group. The symptoms of each group suggest a specific approach to rehabilitation, what to include and, just as important, what to avoid. This section precedes the section on the functional evaluation and therapeutic devices because therapists should first be familiar with the consequences of an individual's eye diseases and realize how the functional outcome affects the program plan for a person with visual impairment.

Cloudy Media

The optical media are responsible for transmitting and focusing light on the macula and retina. A corneal disease, cataracts, an abnormal pupil, or a cloudy vitreous not only cut down the amount of light available to the retina but also scatter light rays to cause glare and haze, which reduces contrast perception. The major effect of these diseases is to cause blurred, hazy vision for distance and reading and to reduce the contrast of objects against their background.

Although cataracts are not in themselves the cause of irremediable low vision, the presence of a cataract may complicate the management of a primary eye disease such as glaucoma, diabetic retinopathy, or macular degeneration. In addition to the visual defects of the primary eye disorder there is added haze, blur, and reduced contrast. Because many levels of disability are experienced with cataracts, not all patients require surgery until the physician feels that visual improvement would be significant and worth the added risk to the success of the procedure. However, often before surgery is recommended, the patient has some degree of difficulty, particularly with lighting. If tests indicate diminished contrast, then the role of lighting and high contrast in the surroundings becomes extremely important, as does a concern for safe, independent mobility.

There may be a problem with lighting in the home for a specific task or glare out of doors. Direct task lighting may have to be redirected at a different angle to avoid surface glare and to provide maximum comfort and visibility. Patients usually prefer the yellow spectrum of incandescent light to the bright white or blue spectrum of halogen or fluorescent lamps. (Halogen as a source of light in a room is acceptable if it is shielded from direct view.) If vision becomes faded or blurred after using any light source for awhile, then the light level may be too high, and a suggested substitution is a lower wattage bulb. Patients also may do well by combining fluorescent ceiling lights with an incandescent lamp at the work surface to offset glare or discomfort that often accompanies exposure to the blue spectrum of fluorescent bulbs.

Another consideration is that, because of glare and poor contrast, magnification may not be as effective as it is in macular disease. Magnification lenses themselves reduce light and decrease contrast.

Sunglasses may be advised for patients who are fine indoors but immediately "blinded" by a sunny day. Selection of the type of filter is best left to an eye care specialist or optician, based on the response of the person to trial lenses, whether Polaroid, yellow, neutral gray or brown tints, or antiglare coatings. The person also can be advised to wear a visor or cap to shield the eyes from overhead light.

Patients may find simple devices helpful: For example, a black matte plastic reading slit (typoscope) placed on a page can reduce the glare of reflected light from shiny paper. Bold-tip pens and black ink can make written material stand out. Important telephone numbers can be listed in large black numbers. Visors reduce overhead glare, even indoors.

A general hint about the use of sunwear as a filter is that gray lenses cut down on light intensity, whereas yellow–brown tints increase contrast. A person may require more than one type of filter depending on the situation.

Central Visual Field Defects (Macular Diseases)

The macula is made up entirely of cones; it comprises a 20° central area in a retina that extends more than 180° horizontally and 60° vertically. This important area is responsible for basic visual functions: detail vision, color vision, daylight vision. Because it is responsible for keen sight, if the macula receptor cells are damaged by atrophy, hemorrhage, laser treatment, or scar tissue, then central vision is reduced. If the damage is extensive, the patient is aware of a blank spot in the center of vision (*scotoma*). The greatest percentage of low vision patients have age-related macular degeneration, and these same patients, who are often at an advanced age, may not only require vision rehabilitation but already be in rehabilitation for an orthopedic problem, poststroke, or some postoperative recovery period.

The loss of vision centrally (either from distortion or a scotoma) calls for an adjustment, usually a spontaneous head or eye turn that shifts the vision away from the center of the macula to the edge (paramacular area). During the period of adaptation, the person with a macular defect learns to look off center ("Do you see better looking up, down, to the right, or to the left?"). Patients may be allowed to look sideways during a therapy session if they see better looking their "own way." Because the visual resolution of this eccentrically located area is less precise, magnified images are needed to interpret that image. Magnifying glasses, such as high power spectacles, hand magnifiers, or stand magnifiers are introduced to allow the person to get used to a magnifying device and, with instruction and repetition, learn to read again. These patients also use nonoptical devices such as bold-tip pens and large-print books and playing cards. When reading becomes a chore, books on tape may be a welcome substitute. Many older people currently are interested in maintaining their computer skills so that they can continue to use electronic mail, see the screen of their Personal Digital Assistant (PDA), and surf the Web. They may need to adapt to using a larger font size, to use magnifying glasses specifically for their computer viewing distance or hand-held device, or to learn the special computer access programs available to people with visual impairments. For an individual with macular degeneration, the provision of low vision aids and suggestions for managing activities of daily living (ADLs) is imperative. Most people are still active and enjoying life, and to them enforced inactivity is unthinkable.

Because the peripheral vision is unaffected (as a rule), individuals with macular disease are able to travel around alone, perhaps using a monocular telescope for signs or, if they prefer, simply asking for directions. They do not usually need special mobility aids such as a cane, unless they need one for support or security. The most difficult activity for independent people to give up is driving. However, the time may come when they must face arranging for alternate types of transportation. This decision must be tactfully but firmly approached—and not at the last minute.

Peripheral Visual Field Defects

When the peripheral retinal vision is obstructed, we lose an aspect of vision that we usually take for granted. Central vision is so important to us that side vision (peripheral visual field) tends to be given a secondary role. However, the peripheral retina provides the orientation clues that result in safe travel. Peripheral vision is a warning system that alerts us to the presence of objects outside the macula, such as landmarks and moving objects (e.g., people, cars). For example, a person cannot drive safely without it, because the peripheral clues keep the car oriented in relation to the rest of the traffic. A person with marked loss of peripheral vision constantly must worry about orientation to the surroundings, about bumping into things, falling, not seeing hazardous situations. The normal peripheral retina is constantly analyzing the environment and directing the macula to look at anything that is either suspicious or needs some form of response action. These patients, no longer relying on this function, accept the mobility cane ("long cane") to explore and map the immediate surroundings for themselves.

Glaucoma

Glaucoma is the most prevalent and most well-known condition in this category. Other important causes of peripheral field loss are retinitis pigmentosa; extensive detached retina after surgery; advanced diabetic retinopathy, including extensive laser photocoagulation for peripheral hemorrhages; and, most important, neurological conditions such as stroke and brain tumor, which have additional physical and cognitive complications.

In regard to glaucoma, it must be emphasized that only in the late stages of decompensation does the glaucoma patient become a low vision patient. The advanced stage of glaucoma is unusual in a patient who has take medication faithfully, although susceptible individuals progress in spite of maximum medication or surgery, especially with so-called *low tension glaucoma.*

The visual field in glaucoma is gradually obliterated, starting in the periphery and gradually advancing toward the macula. As the ganglion cells of the retina drop out, contrast sensitivity gradually decreases until the person loses peripheral awareness and, eventually, macular function. In the late stages of glaucoma, an accurate refraction must be attempted, particularly if the patient has had filtering surgery, which alters the shape of the cornea and thus the refraction of light rays. If reading is still feasible, a low-power hand magnifier may help, with a power of approximately 3x. Nonglare lighting and high-contrast reading and writing aids are helpful. As reading becomes difficult and unresponsive to magnification, traditional magnification aids are no longer effective if there is poor contrast and no healthy peripheral retina. At such a late stage even computer screens are not an option unless a person learns to use voice input, although during the evaluation various aids are always demonstrated. Many of these people must learn nonvisual techniques at a vision rehabilitation agency, such as orientation or mobility instruction and cane or human guide travel, or they can be trained to work with a guide dog. Many older people prefer human guides; some may not have adequate physical strength to manage a dog.

Retinitis Pigmentosa

The remaining central vision in a patient who has retinitis pigmentosa is more useful than the same area in advanced glaucoma. The contrast sensitivity is usually normal. The best devices for individuals with retinitis pigmentosa who desire to do close work are computers (most prefer a computer with clear graphics and simplicity of operation), and closed-circuit television (CCTV) reading machines. Sunglasses that block ultraviolet light and enhance contrast are helpful (Ginsberg, Rosenthal, & Cohen, 1987). Some patients will carry a low power hand magnifier for very small print, but most patients with retinitis pigmentosa benefit from standard distance and reading prescriptions and instruction in cane mobility.

Diabetic Retinopathy

Patients who have *diabetes with retinopathy* are often being treated at the same time for medical problems such as neuropathy, heart condition, stroke, and other circulatory deficits that have to be factored into the rehabilitation plan. Patients may not be able to tolerate much stress; even the act of reading with magnification can be stressful. These patients may be depressed; be taking multiple medications for other systemic problems; and lack energy, which may be interpreted by the therapist as a lack of motivation. Vision may vary from day to day and from morning to afternoon depending on the person's blood glucose level.

Stroke and Brain Injury

The same responses noted in patients with severe diabetes also may be found in people who have sustained brain injuries: fatigue, confusion, depression, and a short attention span. There also may be aphasia and alexia, the inability to read or to interpret the written word, so that simple activities or instructions must be repeated over and over. The most frequent visual field defect in these cases is a hemianopia, either left or right, combined with a hemiplegia. Stroke patients may need prism glasses with the base placed in the direction of the defect. Such a prism may allow the person to overcome the midline (half-field) effect of the hemianopia and to become aware that there is something beyond that midline barrier. Patience, repetition, and involving the family in home therapy are essential, because intensive therapy early in the disease is imperative for progress.

Evaluation Process

A low vision evaluation by an optometrist or ophthalmologist trained in low vision rehabilitation has several objectives: to determine how the specific pathology affects visual function; to quantify several functions; and then, on the basis of the findings, to prescribe devices and suggest or refer that individual for rehabilitation. The evaluation provides essential information for the therapist who will design and implement the treatment plan.

There are many levels of evaluation as well as many approaches to treatment. The ideal approach to vision rehabilitation confirms the diagnosis and applies data from the measurements of functional deficits in visual acuity, refraction, contrast sensitivity, and visual fields to a performance evaluation with optical and nonoptical devices. Each person is different, not only in the extent of the disease but also in the degree of motivation and response. Although there *is* a structured low vision evaluation protocol, there is no such thing as a routine low vision evaluation with a "cookbook" set of directions. Tests can be conducted by anyone, but success depends on their *interpretation*, which must always be matched to the person being evaluated.

Refraction for Best Acuity

A comprehensive evaluation starts with refraction and best-corrected acuity (Rosenthal & Cole, 1996). Vision for distance and near is tested with high-contrast charts. Although the data from these charts are not as significant as contrast data, they verify the refraction and ensure that the person has the best possible vision with standard correction. Chart acuity also is useful to provide baseline vision and to then follow the patient's progress over time.

Central Visual Field

After best acuity is verified, the central visual field is tested using an Amsler grid (see Figure 3.1). The presence of distortion, scotomas, and low-contrast areas in the central (macular) vision is as important as acuity, because defects in the central field affect reading and detail work more so than actual reduction of acuity.

Peripheral Visual Field

A visual field test that measures a person's peripheral field also may be important in some cases. Defects in the peripheral field may affect mobility in disorders such as glaucoma, retinitis pigmentosa neurological brain damage, or diabetic retinopathy. Visual field test results provide information that can suggest the need for mobility instruction. An understanding of an individual's field defects allows the instructor or therapist to anticipate that individual's difficulty locating objects or a problem with orientation in an unfamiliar environment.

As a rule, a printout of an automated field test would be ideal to include in the patient's record, particularly if there is a constricted field that would affect the person's traveling or mobility skills. An understanding of an individual's field defects allows the

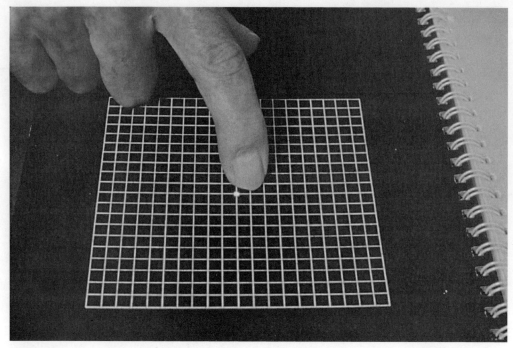

Figure 3.1. The Amsler grid consists of 1-degree squares arranged in a 20-by-20-degree larger square representing the area covered by the entire macula. Macular scotomas can be measured directly. Some patients follow their own progress on a grid.
Photo courtesy of The Lighthouse, Inc. Reprinted with permission.

instructor or therapist to anticipate difficulty locating objects or a problem with orientation in an unfamiliar environment. Because a field test may not always be available, there is a simple and reasonably accurate confrontation field test that can certainly map out gross defects. To map a field, occlude one eye and have the patient look straight ahead at the examiner's opposite eye (patient's left eye looks at examiner's right eye.). Present two fingers at 2, 4, 8, and 10 o'clock, opening and then closing the fingers in each quadrant before moving to the next point, being sure that the patient does not look away, or look at the fingers. That will determine whether any quadrant has a defect or whether the patient has a hemianopia (half of the visual field lost) from brain damage. If the patient does not see fingers in any of the quadrants, that may indicate a constriction. If so, hold two or three fingers in the periphery again at the same hours on the clock, moving the fingers slightly as you approach the center. Note at what distance from the center the person spots the moving fingers. The examiner's eye serves as the normal model. The central field area may be only a few inches in diameter. This is invaluable information in planning a rehabilitation program.

Contrast Sensitivity Testing

Tests of retinal sensitivity are called *contrast sensitivity tests* (they evaluate contrast sensitivity function [CSF]). Contrast sensitivity testing has been used to great advantage in

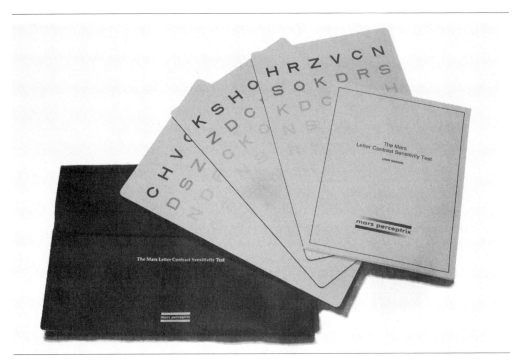

Figure 3.2. A contrast sensitivity test, the Mars Letter Contrast Sensitivity Test, using uniform letters that decrease in sensitivity from close to 100% down to about 1%, measures the percentage of contrast a person has available to function visually.
Photo courtesy of Aries Arditi, PhD, Chappaqua, NY. Reprinted with permission.

vision rehabilitation since 1984, when a study of patients with low vision showed that there was a correlation between response to magnification and CSF (Ginsberg et al., 1987). Responses that fall below the age-related normal level indicate a potentially reduced response to magnification. The lower the score, the more magnification is needed. A very low contrast score warns the clinician that optical magnification may have to be supplanted by electronic instruments (CCTV, computers) that can enlarge print more than an optical lens can. The lowest contrast levels indicate that the rehabilitation must incorporate nonvisual techniques such as cane travel, voice output computers, audiotapes, or Braille.

The diseases that most often reduce the CSF are cataracts, corneal dystrophy, macular degeneration, glaucoma, and diabetic retinopathy. Several tests are available, but the principle of the tests is the same: to measure the eye's ability to discern objects against a background (Bodis-Wollner & Camisa, 1980; see Figure 3.2). Tests in use currently present letters (The Mars Letter Contrast Sensitivity Test, Mars Perceptrix, 1-914-239-3526, http://www.marsperceptrix.com/) or lines in degrees of contrast that provide a measure of an individual's level of contrast perception. These are available from Lighthouse Professional Products at 1-800-826-4200. The macula is the structure that is most sensitive to degrees of contrast, but the parafoveal retina (next to the macula) and the peripheral retina also are sensitive enough to provide useful vision when the macula has been damaged.

Once the diagnosis, correct refraction and function tests have been completed, the rehabilitation planning can begin. The next section considers aspects of vision rehabilitation that help the patient work with the devices whose power and type have been suggested by the evaluation. Advantages and disadvantages are described for various types of devices. The next section also deals with the instruction process and the modification of devices and techniques that may be necessary as the patient learns new skills and becomes more knowledgeable and selective.

Low Vision Optical and Adaptive Devices: Functional Considerations

In the course of the low vision evaluation, before introducing devices to the patient, the examiner has considered the pathology and its effects on the patient's ability to perform. The function tests have been analyzed, the power of the devices has been calculated, and the devices are now introduced in relation to functional capacity and task objectives. Each patient has interests, level of motivation, intelligence, a coping history, and complex intangibles that must now be considered. Once the devices are selected, the patient must learn and apply adaptation skills, whether reading with magnifiers, using a computer, or a closed-circuit reading machine. Skill continues to grow with practice.

Basic devices for low vision are either optical, such as magnifying lenses, telescopes, and sunglasses; electronic, such as special computers and CCTV; or nonoptical, such as reading stands, lighting, writing aids, and travel aids (Williams, 1996).

Spectacles

Magnifying lenses, when mounted in spectacle frames, must be used at a specific distance dictated by the power of the lens. The stronger the lens, the closer the reading material is held to the glass, that is, 13 in (33 cm) or less, often as close as 2 or 3 in (5 or 7 cm). Both hands are involved with holding reading material if it is not mounted on a reading stand. Because of the optical limitation of magnifying lenses, patients who read with both eyes must be helped converge at such a close reading distance by the incorporation of base-in prisms in the reading lenses (see Figure 3.3). Patients who use only one eye use a single lens but also must hold the print at the focal distance of the lens.

Focal distance in centimeters is related to the dioptric strength of the lens using the following formula: focal length (f) equals 100 divided by the dioptric strength (D), or $f = 100 / D$. For example, a 10 diopter lens would have a working distance (f) of 100 over $10 = 10$ cm. To convert to inches, divide the number of centimeters by 2.5, in this case, $10 / 2.5 = 4$ in.

A lamp should be positioned in front of the face so that light falls directly onto the page without creating glare. The person has to read slowly, usually one word at a time at first, and to move the paper evenly past the eye. Some patients can scan by moving their

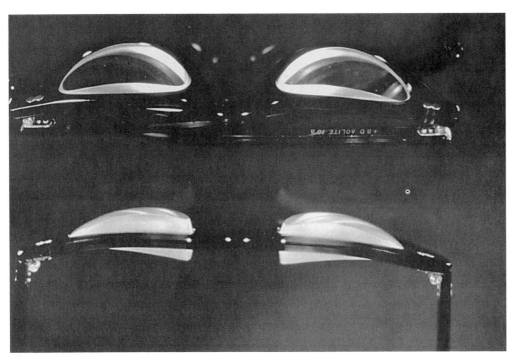

Figure 3.3. Base-in prism glasses allow a person with a visual impairment to read with strong magnifying lenses at a distance closer than 10 inches. Prisms reduce the eye strain that would otherwise occur with reading with strong magnifying glasses.
Photo courtesy of The Lighthouse, Inc. Reprinted with permission.

heads, although this is more difficult and takes hours of practice. The advantages of a spectacle lens compared with a handheld lens are that the reading field is wider, which allows greater reading speed, and both hands can be used to hold the reading material. Preference varies depending on the person's interest in reading and the degree of macular damage. With advanced loss, many prefer a handheld or stand-mounted magnifier. If the disease involves peripheral field loss, a spectacle may not be appropriate because an image close to the eye is larger than the available central field. With macular degeneration, the patient has the entire peripheral retina available for magnified vision.

Hand Magnifiers

Most patients, regardless of their eye condition, will use a handheld magnifier for a variety of short-term tasks. A handheld lens is held away from the eye, which increases the work space between the eye and lens (see Figure 3.4). For most patients, the increase in working distance is more comfortable than the closer distance required by spectacle lenses. A first step for some patients is to practice doing small practical tasks, such as reading a stove dial and microwave settings, finding a television station, or setting a thermostat. Although patients traditionally use magnifiers for shopping and reading mail, labels, menus, and recipes, many learn to read text efficiently, although scanning at a slower pace than with spectacles.

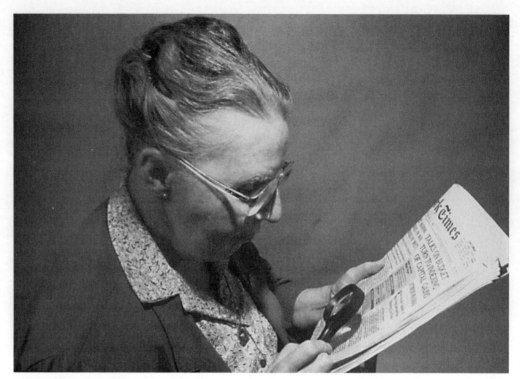

Figure 3.4. A handheld magnifying lens allows low vision patients to hold material farther away from their eyes than required by an equally strong spectacle lens. Many older patients find it easier to read in this posture.
Photo courtesy of The Lighthouse, Inc. Reprinted with permission.

For many patients, starting with a hand magnifier as a training device allows them eventually to adjust to spectacles. Patients also may use a hand magnifier with their ordinary spectacles to gain a little more magnification for specific tasks. Patients with peripheral field loss prefer to use a low-power hand magnifier, which enhances but does not enlarge the image so much that it disappears into the lost field area.

For patients with tremors or orthopedic or neurological deficits, hand magnifiers are probably not the aid of choice. Stand magnifiers are sturdier and easier to hold.

Hand magnifiers can be illuminated or nonilluminated and are available in a wide range of powers. They are available from Lighthouse Professional Products at-1-800-826-4200, or Independent Living Aids at http:www.independentliving.com.

Stand Magnifiers

A stand magnifier can be thought of as a hand magnifier mounted on a base that rests on a page. Patients who cannot hold a hand magnifier steadily should be presented with the same power in a stand. Its base holds the lens close to its focal distance so that the patient does not have to struggle to maintain the working distance. This premounted lens is stable and easy to maneuver for patients with a tremor or arthritic hands. Many stands have

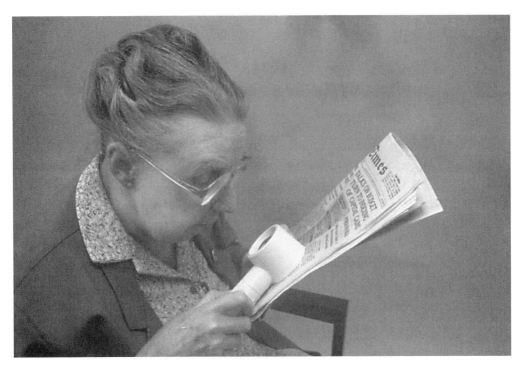

Figure 3.5. A stand magnifier helps patients with tremors hold a magnifier supported directly on the page. Some stands have internal light sources that enhance reading.
Photo coutesy of The Lighthouse, Inc. Reprinted with permission.

built-in illumination, which makes them the aid of choice for those patients who also need an extra light source. Stand magnifiers are also available in nonilluminated and illuminated form. Many stands now are equipped with long-life LED bulbs so that batteries are less of an expense and do not require so much upkeep. Many patients with glaucoma prefer to use the illuminated stands not only because of the light but also for the ease of maintaining focus (see Figure 3.5).

Telescopes

The telescope tends to be overemphasized in vision rehabilitation, although to many people it is synonymous with low vision because it is dramatic and charismatic. It not only looks as if it were special, but it also has a unique optical characteristic that no other device has: the capacity to focus at any distance, from infinity to very near. Of particular importance is the intermediate or arm's-length work distance, which is beyond the visual range of any of the other devices and focuses at an important range in daily life: shelves in the market and library, display cases, computer screens, home repairs, foot care, and playing music.

Telescopes are most frequently prescribed as handeld monoculars, but they also can be mounted in a spectacle frame to free both hands (see Figure 3.6). Because of their light

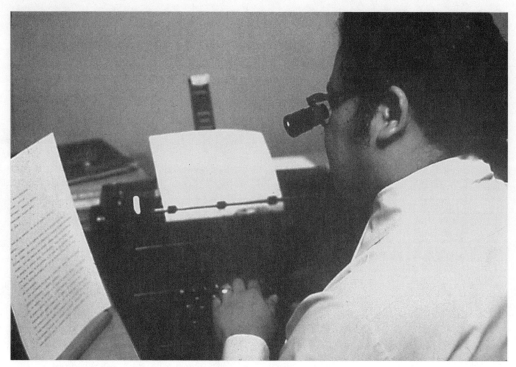

Figure 3.6. Telescopes are infrequently prescribed, but for many patients, seeing street signs, looking for a bus or taxi, or watching a stage performance are important activities. Patients have to be instructed in the correct way to focus and use a telescope.
Photo courtesy of The Lighthouse, Inc. Reprinted with permission.

weight, spectacle-mounted telescopes may be preferable to heavy binoculars for use in museums, movies, lectures, and art exhibits. Before computer programs were available in enlarged type, telescopes were prescribed for reading a computer screen, but they were never ideal because of the decreased illumination and small field. For students in school, seeing the board may warrant the prescription of a spectacle-mounted telescope.

Aside from cost, telescopic devices have two optical disadvantages: (a) a restricted field no more than a few inches in width and (b) little flexibility or depth of focus in terms of the working distance. Telescopes also have a cosmetic disadvantage: They are very conspicuous and call attention to a person's disability, which may not be desirable. Telescopes in a frame also block out the surroundings when the patient is looking through them, which could represent a hazard in mobility unless special instruction is included in the rehabilitation. Most patients prefer a handheld monocular that can be used as needed and is relatively inconspicuous.

Closed-Circuit Television

Reproducing reading material in a range of font sizes with a CCTV camera and monitor is another alternative to low vision reading lenses. Several options are available with closed-circuit reading machines and can be found in the Lighthouse Professional

Products catalog. It is possible to sit at a normal distance from the screen, moving the reading material by hand under the television camera on a movable x–y table, or to use a smaller handheld camera to scan the reading material. Some devices are battery powered so that they may be taken to school or to a library in a briefcase.

Most patients choose high-contrast white or yellow letters on a dark background, but most CCTV sets now include several other choices in terms of font size, color, and other options. CCTV provides the greatest range of magnification (up to 60x) and the best contrast of any optical device so, for patients who need high contrast to read, the CCTV is the best choice.

Other Techniques in Rehabilitation

ADLs encompass many mundane tasks for which magnification with optical devices is not necessary. Part of the rehabilitation will emphasize such simple maneuvers as sitting closer to a television or to a person to see details more clearly and using objects that are designed with enlarged letters or numbers, such as on clock faces, telephones, timers, large-print books, and computer programs (Williams, 1996).

The myriad daily tasks, such as shopping, cooking, and personal care, can be more frustrating than the inability to read a book because they have become time consuming, and the patient's performance is less competent than in former days. Suggestions to help the patient adapt more efficiently include marking objects such as seasonings and medications with large-print or tactile labels and arranging items in an orderly fashion in drawers, closets, kitchens, and bathrooms. Patients should be encouraged to use auditory skills, to explore options for themselves, and to think during their rehabilitation about realistic priorities as they work with the therapist evolving new approaches to old skills.

Summary

Concerns about an aging population will escalate as longevity becomes the rule rather than the exception. Any professional involved with geriatric caregiving is faced with the recognition that, at some point, normal aging changes become pathology. Decision making and program planning are related to a person's functional status. However, eye care, instead of including vision rehabilitation, has traditionally relied on conventional eyeglasses, medical treatment, or surgery. Only a limited segment of the aging population has had access to vision rehabilitation. The prospective increase in the aging population and subsequent demand for low vision care may change the current attitude of inertia within the eye care professions, as well as increase knowledge about the eyes in other specialties and for other rehabilitation professionals. Legislation has been pending for years to include coverage for vision rehabilitation offered by certified low vision therapists, rehabilitation teachers, and orientation or mobility instructors under Medicare, although occupational therapists have been included in coverage for medical-based rehabilitation for decades.

People with visual challenges who are part of the upcoming geriatric generation are not going to be satisfied with the platitude that "nothing can be done," because it is obvious that a combination of a low vision evaluation and prescription of low vision adaptive devices, with thorough training in their application, combined with other rehabilitation techniques, will maintain optimum quality of visual function for patients who develop low vision.

References

Arditi, A. (2002). *Color contrast*. New York: Lighthouse International.

Ball, K., Owsley, C., & Beard, B. (1989). Clinical visual perimetry underestimates peripheral field problems in older adults. *Clinical Vision Sciences, 4,* 229–249.

Bodis-Wollner, I., & Camisa, J. M. (1980). Contrast sensitivity measurement in clinical diagnosis. In G. Lassell & J. T. W. Van Dalen (Eds.), *Neurophthalmology* (Vol. 1, pp. 373–401). Princeton, NJ: Excerpta Medica.

Faye, E. E. (1996). Pathology and visual function. In B. P. Rosenthal, R. G. Cole, & R. London (Eds.), *Functional assessment of low vision* (pp. 63–75). St. Louis, MO: Mosby.

Faye, E. E. (2000). Poor vision. In J. C. Evans, B. L. Beattie, J. P. Michel, & G. K. Wilcox (Eds.), *Oxford text of geriatric medicine* (pp. 881–893). New York: Oxford University Press.

Faye, E. E. (2003). Low vision. In D. Vaughan, T. Asbury, & P. Riordan-Eva (Eds.), *General ophthalmology* (16th ed., pp. 405–412). Norwalk, CT: Appleton & Lange.

Ginsburg, A. P., Rosenthal, B., & Cohen, J. (1987). The evaluation of reading capability of low vision patients using the Vision Contrast Test System (VCTS). In G. C. Woo (Ed.), *Low vision: Principles and application* (pp. 17–18). New York: Springer-Verlag.

Hemenger, R. P. (1984). Intraocular light scatter in normal vision loss with age. *Applied Optics, 23,* 1972–1974.

Hofstetter, H. W. (1965). A longitudinal study of amplitude changes in presbyopia. *American Journal of Optometry, 42,* 3–8.

Liebowitz, H. M., Krueger, D. E., Maunder, L. R., et al. (1980). The Framingham Eye Study monograph. *Survey of Ophthalmology, 24*(Suppl.), 335–610.

Lighthouse Professional Products catalog 2004. 1-800-826-4200.

Marmor, M. F. (1995). Normal age-related vision changes and their effect on vision. In E. E. Faye & C. C. Stuen (Eds.), *The aging eye and low vision (A study guide)* (pp. 6–10). New York: Lighthouse International.

Owsley, C., Sekuler, R., & Siemsen, D. (1983). Contrast sensitivity throughout adulthood. *Vision Research, 23,* 689–699.

Owsley, C., & Sloan, M. E. (1980). Contrast sensitivity, acuity, and the perception of real world targets. *British Journal of Ophthalmology Vision Sciences, 19,* 401–406.

Rosenthal, B. P., & Cole, R.G. (Eds.). (1996). *Functional assessment of low vision*. St. Louis, MO: Mosby.

Williams, D. R. (1996). Functional adaptive devices. In B. P. Rosenthal & R. G. Cole (Eds.), *Remediation and management of low vision* (pp. 71–121). St. Louis, MO: Mosby.

Wolf, E. (1960). Glare and age. *Archives of Ophthalmology, 64,* 502–514.

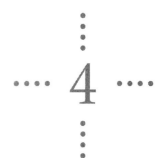

Visual Rehabilitation of the Neurologically Involved Person

Maureen Connor, OTR/L

William V. Padula, OD, FAAO, FNOR

The underlying theme of occupational therapy, frequently reinforced during the schooling of therapists, is one of *holism*. Holism is the process of treating the whole person and choosing therapeutic activities that have specific personal meaning to the patient. This approach to treatment is the cornerstone of the profession. Yet it has been the observation of the authors that, in the face of the ever-changing, rapid-paced, and time-limited health care system, some clinicians resort to reductionistic views that limit seeing the patient as a whole person.

Health care clinicians in general have felt the need to reduce their focus and define specialties specifically to accommodate the complexity of the human body. The need for reductionism for detailed study and scientific understanding is evident. However, it is essential to continue to view the human system or systems as wholes, as the complexity of physiology gives us reason to believe that systems are somehow greater than their parts.

It is this perspective that requires the visual–perceptual function of the patient with neurological impairments be viewed in light of all the other systems with which it interacts. The observation of the authors is that occupational therapists frequently do not focus enough on the profound relationship of vision and function. In general, optometrists and ophthalmologists tend to concentrate exclusively on oculomotor function and the health of the eyeball, optic nerve, and visual cortex. Both of these views demonstrate inherent limitations when attempting to assess the functional behavioral impairments of patients with posthead injury.

This chapter presents the following: a working model of the visual process, a brief definition of neuro-optometric rehabilitation, the symptomatology of posttrauma vision syndrome (PTVS) and visual midline shift syndrome (VMSS), treatment approaches of both optometrists and therapists, some case examples, and some conclusions.

Central and Ambient Visual Processes: A Working Model of Vision

A model of vision as divided into two processes—the central and the ambient—will help qualify the further discussion of the interaction between vision and function. This model is described by Trevarthen (1968) and Leibowitz and Post (1982). The central or focal visual process involves that which we classically think of as seeing in both the real and anatomical senses. Through this focal system, the object of focalization, that is, the object being attended to, is seen in detail with acuity and color perception. Neurologically, the central processing begins at the macula, which is composed of cone cells responsible for high resolution and color detection, and progresses to the central areas of the visual cortex through the optic nerve. In contrast, spatial awareness and detection of movement are the primary purposes of the ambient system. The ambient process interrelates with the central visual process by providing the peripheral awareness required for a reference environment or background. This will spatially orient both the object of focus and the perceiver's body in space.

Many nerve cells originating from the eye send collateral fibers to other areas of the brain before reaching the highly organized seeing area in the cortex (see Figure 4.1). Trevarthen (1968) has concluded that the dorsal ganglion of the lateral geniculate body may function as an integrating center in addition to its role as a relay and distribution center. This means that the lateral geniculate is important for the relay of visual information to portions of the brain other than the visual cortex. The lateral geniculate body actively responds to diffuse illumination and any movement of light across the retina. Cortical cells respond to detail as well as specific axes of illumination on the retina. Ganglion cells emanate from the retina through the optic nerve and optic chiasm to the optic tract, where all the fibers synapse at the lateral geniculate body. At this point, axons are directed to the pretectal nucleus (pupillary constriction) and the superior colliculus, which importantly becomes related to posture, movement, and orientation to position in space (Wolfe, 1968). The superior colliculus receives fibers from the optic tract via the superior brachium and occipital cortex via the optic radiations through the lateral geniculate and from the spinotectal tract connecting it with sensorimotor information from the spinal cord and medulla.

The Ambient Visual System and the Sensorimotor Feedback Loop

The ambient visual process links with and becomes part of the sensorimotor feedback loop at the level of the midbrain. The matching of information that occurs between the ambient

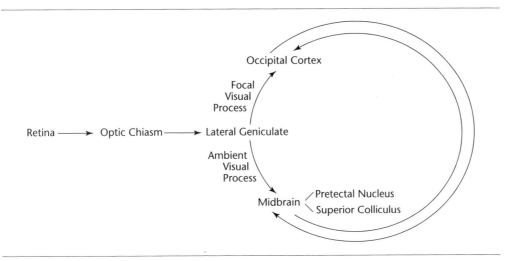

Figure 4.1. Neurological relationship of vision to occipital cortex and midbrain.

visual process and the kinesthetic, proprioceptive, vestibular, and tactile systems sets up a spatial framework that becomes the basis of higher sensory interpretation. The sensorimotor feedback loop involving the midbrain provides a feed-forward system to areas of higher cortical function through receiving as well as sending fiber tracts to the occipital, temporal, parietal, and frontal cortexes (Nelson & Benabib, 1992). The superior colliculus receives a large quantity of axons in relationship to vision. Without the matching of information that occurs between the ambient process (including the vestibular ocular reflex) and the other portions of the sensorimotor feedback system, we would actually perceive an image as jumping and moving about each time we made a shift of our eyes or our body (Padula, 1996). The midbrain is responsible for providing information to the visual cortex about aligning and developing integration of the central images from both eyes.

Posttrauma Vision Syndrome

This working model for vision provides us with a perspective through which we can begin to assess and treat the functional deficits observed in patients with traumatic brain injury (TBI), cerebrovascular accident (CVA), or other neurological disorders. Those optometrists who have observed the functional behaviors of these patients and are treating the visual process with techniques that have been specifically found to be beneficial to this population have developed a specialty termed neuro-optometric rehabilitation. Optometrists practicing this specialty and other clinicians working in the field of neurologic rehabilitation have observed consistencies in the visual and motoric symptomatology of this population. PTVS as defined by Padula, Argyris, and Ray (1994) presents with consistent characteristics and symptoms.

Common characteristics include

- Exotropia or high exophoria
- Low blink rate

- Convergence insufficiency
- Poor fixations and pursuits
- Accommodative dysfunction
- Unstable ambient vision
- Spatial disorientation
- Increased myopia.

Common symptoms include

- Possible diplopia
- Staring behavior
- Poor visual memory
- Perceived movement of print or stationary objects
- Asthenopia
- Photophobia
- Poor concentration and attention.

The introduction of a theory postulating an explanation for the above characteristics of PTVS is relevant here as a prerequisite to further discussion of observed functional behaviors and appropriate treatments. Dysfunction in the ambient visual process at the level of the midbrain (mechanism described above) following a TBI may contribute to the observable visual as well as perceptual, cognitive, and motoric deficits. The ambient process normally provides stabilization and orientation of the external visual world. Neurological damage disrupts spatial awareness, causing distortion of temporal and spatial concepts.

Exophoria as a Characteristic of PTVS

To understand the effect of a perceptually based spatial dysfunction on eye posture, we first review normal eye postures. *Convergence* is the turning in of the eyes to view a near object. *Divergence* is the turning out of the eyes to observe an image further away. *Exophoria* is the tendency for both eyes to align on a point in space further than the object of intended focus or the tendency for one or both eyes to drift outward on a cover test. A cover test requires that one eye of the patient be covered by the examiner during the act of having the patient look at an object with both eyes. Normally, the covered eye maintains posture toward the object of regard. In the case of an exophoria, the eyes deviate outward upon being covered. The difference between exophoria and exotropia is that in the latter an actual deviation of one eye outward is exhibited. As described earlier, the balance between the focal and ambient processes is mediated by sensorimotor feedback. Eye posture can be used as a barometer of this balance. An imbalance between those processes causes the spatial distortion of an expansion of central space with a relative compression of peripheral space. This spatial distortion promotes objects appearing to the perceiver to be farther away with a concurrent exophoria or exotropia noted. It is, therefore, postulated that this spatial distortion mediates the behavior of exophoria and other difficulties with binocularity, rather than the other way around.

A further description of the concept of spatial distortion may assist readers here. Think of a three-dimensional face with the closest point to you being the tip of a big nose. Notice all the contours of the face spatially, what is further away and what is closer, what is more central to the face and what is more lateral. Now imagine the face made of putty in your hands. If peripheral space were expanded equally on either side of the head, with a relative compression of central space and with only so much space that the face can occupy, this would cause the face to flatten from the sides as if you were pressing in the putty ears. Notice what this does to the face, moving the tip of the nose closer to you and flattening the face in the lateral to medial plane. Now try expanding space centrally, with a relative compression of peripheral space, causing the face to flatten front to back, as if you are pressing in at the nose and the back of the head. Relatively speaking, if the nose were your point of regard again, it would move farther away from you and the face would eventually appear flat, or more two-dimensional, taking up more space centrally and appearing wider. This is a simplification; however, it begins to ground the concept of spatial distortion.

As previously stated, exophoria is a common characteristic of PTVS. It is easier now to appreciate how an expansion of central space is concurrent with an exophoria or exotropia. To simplify, central space flattens and expands, while peripheral space becomes relatively compressed. The exophoria, in this case, is a result of the mismatch of information caused by this distortion and not a cause in itself.

Convergence Insufficiency, Accommodative Spasm, and Time–Space Dysfunction as Characteristics of PTVS

Convergence is the ability of the eyes to come together to fuse the image of objects at near. According to this theory, convergence insufficiency is noted as a by-product of spatial distortion, originating from the imbalance between the ambient and focal visual processing systems, not as an oculomotor deficit in and of itself. Again, the perceptual mismatch causing the eyes to deviate outward will be concurrent with a convergence insufficiency or difficulty with bringing eyes inward to focalize at near.

Because of a flattening of space on the near to far axis, as described above, depth perception is impaired and temporal relationships are disturbed. As an example, a ball coming toward the person will appear to become larger but not necessarily moving through an accurate representation of space. Suddenly, the ball will appear to speed up when it reaches the zone of space that the person perceives more accurately (i.e., that which has not been perceptually flattened). Secondary to this perceptual mismatch, far space tends to be conceptually lost and an overfocalization at near occurs, causing the patient to present with an accommodative spasm, that is stuck at near, or an inability to accommodate or focus on far images and a tendency, therefore, toward myopia or near-sightedness. On the face of it, this may appear to readers to be a contradiction to the above-described exophoria when viewed in traditional oculomotor terms. However, myopia as described here can be thought of as an overfocalization as compensation for a high exophoria or exotropia to prevent diplopia (see below). In other words, in working hard to fuse the image, a compensatory near focus causes accommodative spasm at near and myopia. Again, the problems of binocularity are not the place of origin of the perceptual motor mismatching, but the result of the process of spatial distortion related to dysfunction in the ambient system as described above.

Double Vision as a Characteristic of PTVS

Diplopia (blurred or double vision) often results from the deviated eye posture and convergence insufficiency described above. Where in space the object of regard is when diplopia is experienced depends on the severity of spatial distortion and subsequent degree of convergence and fusion insufficiency. When the ambient visual process, which normally assists in organizing and orienting the images from both eyes (through the information it receives from kinesthetic, proprioceptive, and vestibular centers), is disrupted by neurological damage, diplopia can occur related to visual spatial disorientation.

Attention and Cognitive Deficits as Related to PTVS

Highly intense focalization or an overattention to objects of detail tends to be the compensation for a highly confusing perceptual world. It is also the natural result of an expansion of central space with a relative disregard for peripheral spatial awareness. A relationship has been observed, not only between these perceptual distortions and visual motor mismatching (causing changes in muscle tonus, coordination, balance, and posture) but also between vision and cognition.

To assist in concretizing the relationship between the visual–perceptual process and cognition, it may be helpful for readers to think of how one internalizes visual space (i.e., in the mind's eye) to think about and understand concepts. It has been demonstrated through repeated observation and interview that people encode their experiences or memories through specific, predictable visual parameters or submodalities (Bandler, 1985) such as quality or amount of light, amount of movement, or size of the picture (the picture in one's head as the experience is being recalled). In other words, one person might prioritize the importance of past experiences by the amount of light in the picture when remembered, and another might do this through the size or panoramic quality of it. This is a process the mind does without conscious awareness but can be retrieved consciously when intended.

This concept is introduced only to assist readers in understanding cognition in visual terms. It is from this perspective that various measures of cognition, for example, attention, memory, and mental flexibility, can be discussed.

Readers may note how one attends to one object, concept, or picture in internal visual space by arranging or knowing where that object fits spatially or in relationship to other objects or concepts, that is, when thinking about the object of attention, it may tend to be placed more centrally for immediate attention, while related concepts may be placed peripherally. Other unrelated concepts are off the screen entirely, so to speak. An analogy for those who have used computers is the program Windows® one can call many related documents to the screen at one time with some made smaller, others larger, depending on present focus. Another way of demonstrating this is that people who talk with their hands are frequently showing their internal representation of ideas in space (again, in the mind's eye) by where they place that idea in space with their hands.

Given this model, readers may begin to predict what may occur in the case of a patient who has experienced a TBI. If external spatial concepts are distorted (as described above under the beginning description of PTVS), an amplification of central space with a flattening of depth may conceptually correlate with all objects of regard (objects of present cognitive attention) having equal rate with little control over placing objects of intended focus in an internal spatial place of importance or priority. This visual–cognitive correlation or parallel relates to the behavior initially observed with those coming out of coma at Ranchos level 4 or 5, as an example. Many clinicians have observed that external stimulation at this point in recovery must be reduced and introduced in a graded manner to promote understanding and reduce agitated behavior. It is as if all information is equal with no filtering mechanism. In visual terms, this attention disorder is similar to having all external stimuli overlapping in the central field in the same place, with little ability to sort or prioritize for attentional strategies.

One can only assume that this individual would begin to attempt to cope with this experience. Because the perceptual–cognitive distortions still coexist, one barometer clinicians can observe regarding this coping is the overfocalization process. Objects are conceptually spread out, and then space is pulled in from a panorama of objects or concepts that appear to have no relationship to each other to a single object of focus that is singled out at any given time with a required relative disregard for the periphery of objects around it. Attention deficits noted in those who have had TBI stem from both the former and latter mechanisms, that is, first, no filtering mechanism and second, overfocalization as a coping strategy. The former promotes confusion regarding where to attend, while the latter causes an overattention to one object of regard with a relative inattention to others. Clinicians may note this transition as behavioral change from the agitated, confused behavior of RLA Scale Level 4 to the cognitive inflexibility of RLA Scale Levels 5–7.

Overfocalization correlates to concrete thinking as one idea or concept is overemphasized without adequate comparison to those ideas related to or affecting that concept. Many people may relate to a time when under stress they thought they knew a solution to a problem and sped down the trajectory of that one solution analogous to a super highway, disregarding contradictory information or better solutions popping up in the periphery in the form of exit signs. This is a very mild example of what patients with TBI experience and why they are often noted to be adverse to change. Too much movement literally and figuratively is quite challenging to the accompanying strategy of overfocalization.

This tendency toward overattention to one object or concept visually and cognitively also relates to a cognitive behavior often demonstrated by patients with TBI termed *perseveration*. Frequently, verbal clients will state the same worry or idea repeatedly saying, "I can't get it off my mind." Those around them often say, "Why can't you just put that in the back of your mind?" Notice the words used and remember the analogy of the computer screen. Another fear of patients with TBI is that once they let it go, the idea will not be able to be retrieved from memory, a result of overattention to a new concept.

Impaired memory post-TBI correlates to aforementioned attentional deficits, as memory requires adequate attention for the encoding process. Also, neurologically the mechanism to encode memories (as described above) may be disrupted.

Other Symptoms of PTVS

Observable staring behavior is related to the symptoms reviewed thus far: staring can be related to either general inattention or the locking in process of overattention to one idea or object.

Overfocalization represents another attempt at stabilizing a visual world that may appear to move. As described above, the ambient system is believed to be responsible for stabilizing an image so that it does not appear to move when the eyes, head, or body move. Frequently, those who have had a TBI experience their external world as moving or print as jumping around as they attempt to read. Those whose cognition is too impaired to make sense of the movement often make sense of it in other ways, which may be somewhat inaccurately termed as hallucinations, such as seeing snakes or bugs crawling on the walls. Smooth pursuits and saccades are interrupted both by the instability of the visual world and the compensatory overfocalization. This overfocalization while reading is like reading with tunnel vision or with a magnifying glass. Overattention or "locking in" on one word or set of words without the overall reference picture of the other words limits the ability to find the next word to read and, most notably, to connect the words to make meaning, reducing reading comprehension.

Visual instability and spatial distortion, as described, very much affect and interrelate with gross and fine motor coordination, balance, posture, and imbalances in muscle tonus. Muscle tonus may be increased around the head, neck, and thoracic regions when

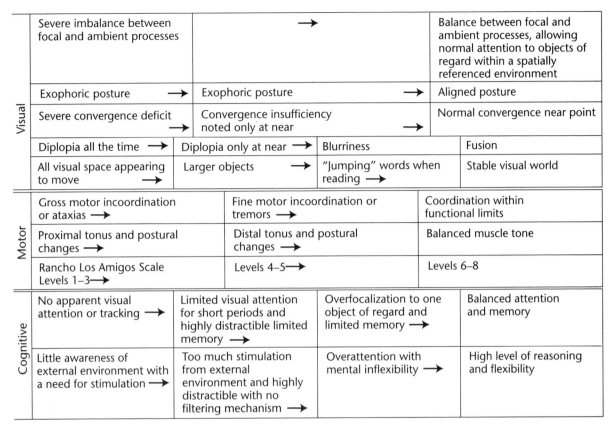

Visual	Severe imbalance between focal and ambient processes	→		Balance between focal and ambient processes, allowing normal attention to objects of regard within a spatially referenced environment
	Exophoric posture →	Exophoric posture →		Aligned posture
	Severe convergence deficit →	Convergence insufficiency noted only at near →		Normal convergence near point
	Diplopia all the time →	Diplopia only at near →	Blurriness	Fusion
	All visual space appearing to move →	Larger objects →	"Jumping" words when reading →	Stable visual world
Motor	Gross motor incoordination or ataxias →	Fine motor incoordination or tremors →		Coordination within functional limits
	Proximal tonus and postural changes →	Distal tonus and postural changes →		Balanced muscle tone
	Rancho Los Amigos Scale Levels 1–3→	Levels 4–5→		Levels 6–8
Cognitive	No apparent visual attention or tracking →	Limited visual attention for short periods and highly distractible limited memory →	Overfocalization to one object of regard and limited memory →	Balanced attention and memory
	Little awareness of external environment with a need for stimulation →	Too much stimulation from external environment and highly distractible with no filtering mechanism →	Overattention with mental inflexibility →	High level of reasoning and flexibility

Figure 4.2. Parallel between functional systems.
Note. Arrows indicate continuum from severe deficits or just post-injury through recovery.
Created by M. Connor.

the visual system is stressed. The example of the ball given earlier to demonstrate disturbed temporal spatial relationships helps to explain observed incoordination and perceptual motor mismatching. During the complete evaluation, the effect of disturbances of the visual process as well as of motor components requires consideration. Figure 4.2 serves as a summary and an overview for use with a thorough assessment of a neurologically impaired patient. Please note that these are generalizations only, and many exceptions may exist.

Interventions for PTVS

Now that readers have become familiar with the behavioral symptoms of PTVS and the authors' theory of the cause of these symptoms, it is satisfying to present treatment ideas that appear to be consistently helpful with this visual syndrome. Two of these treatments are base-in prism and binasal occlusion. Two diopters base-in prism ground into prescription lenses have been observed to effectively decrease the visual stress and therefore the symptomatology described above. The base side of prisms compress space, therefore, both prisms base-in will compress central space and relatively amplify peripheral space to assist in remediating the spatial distortion described above. The base-in prism counters the expansion of central space and the compression of peripheral space. It creates a relative balance between the focal and ambient processes, in turn affecting visual, motor, and cognitive function.

Binasal occlusion is a treatment technique whereby translucent tape is placed over a person's lenses, partially occluding the nasal portion of the visual field. This technique may further reduce stress in the ambient system both by filtering out some of the visual information and by providing a vertical line by which visual space can be organized, much the same way one might grab a pole on the subway to stabilize oneself. Research (Padula, Argyris, & Ray, 1994) using base-in prism and binasal occlusion on people with TBI demonstrated with *visual evoked potentials* (VEPs) that the binocular symptoms observed following TBI are not oculomotor in origin but are a result of interference in the ambient visual process at the level of the midbrain. This research showed a correlation between an increase in the VEP amplitudes and the use of binasal occluders on those with TBI. The control group showed a decrease in amplitude. The amplitudes of VEP (brain waves produced by the occipital cortex) appear to be highly influenced by the ambient visual process. Dysfunction of the ambient visual process such as found after a TBI reduces the amplitude of the VEP for people with PTVS. As proposed earlier, the ambient visual process is an integrative process involving vision, kinesthetic, proprioceptive, and vestibular feedback. Therefore, in addition to incorporating neuro-optometric interventions, such as base-in prism and binasal occlusion, therapists and optometrists alike should incorporate such integrative approaches as neurodevelopmental treatment, proprioceptive neuromuscular facilitation, and sensory integration to assist in concurrently influencing the motor and ambient visual systems. The information relayed to the ambient visual system through weight bearing, challenging righting reflexes, vestibular activities, reaching activities, and tactile activities is essential to the remediation of the visual spatial awareness required for effective focalization. Because focalization is the system most immediately understood as traditional seeing, the focus in evaluation and treatment of vision all too often is the mechanism of focalization in the eyeball and the immediate visual cortex. Therefore, the authors propose that neuromuscular reeducation in combination with optometric intervention is the most effective treatment approach.

Hemianopsia and Visual Inattention

Evaluation and treatment will be further addressed after the following discussion of other types of perceptual and spatial distortions observed in patients who are post-CVA, head trauma, and so forth. Once readers have a complete perspective of the theories presented here, a discussion of treatment will be more relevant.

Any clinician who has worked with patients post-CVA or other neurological event has observed that these patients frequently present with some form of visual–perceptual deficit; some are immediately observable in any context, others only while functioning in certain distracting environments. However, the common link is that these deficits are quite influential in the patients functioning, often disturbing activities of daily living (ADL), coordination, posture, attention, reading, and figure–ground tasks.

Visual–perceptual neglect or inattention and visual field deficits (most commonly homonymous hemianopsia) are common deficits noted post-CVA. The former presents as an inattention or decreased perceptual awareness of a portion of visual space, the latter as an actual visual field loss, that is, not being able to see a portion of visual space. A homonymous hemianopsia occurs when vision is lost in the nasal portion of one eye and the temporal portion of the other, causing an inability to see in half of the visual field. These deficits may be observed by therapists in a more formal screening or in behavioral assessment. If a patient is able to verbalize and attend adequately, visual fields may be generally assessed by sitting in front of the patient with his or her eyes focused on the practitioner's face, holding long dowels with colored tips at arm's length behind the patient's head. Bringing the dowels into different quadrants of the periphery, the practitioner asks the patient to report when he or she sees the dowels come into view in the periphery. This should be performed both binocularly and monocularly (by covering one eye). Any test like this may make apparent other deficits like decreased visual attention, dysfunctional level of distractibility, and impaired immediate memory. A perceptual neglect may be observed by standing behind the patient with one dowel positioned on each side of the head, quickly placing and removing one dowel into the periphery on the right or left side or both sides, and asking the patient to indicate seeing on the left, right, or both. If the patient consistently misses one side when one or both are introduced, an inattention to that side is possible.

Patients can present with one or both of these deficits (i.e., visual field loss or visual field neglect). The distinction between the two can often be noted behaviorally when objective measures are difficult to complete because of cognitive–linguistic dysfunction. With a visual field loss, frequently searching behavior is noted when the patient is attempting to locate an object of intended focus. In the case of an inattention or neglect, the object of focus is found more quickly when using other senses as reinforcing anchors to the image, such as a person's voice or having the patient touch the object of regard. Behaviors such as running into the wall while walking or propelling a wheelchair, reading or writing on only one side of the page, and not locating objects on one side when performing functional tasks can be indicative of one or both of these deficits. It is important to note that patients with milder deficits may only demonstrate them under personal stress or in stressful environments. For example, a patient may demonstrate a high-level neglect while in a grocery store by being unable to locate certain objects on the left side of the aisle.

These deficits have thus far been presented primarily from a visual perspective. It is instructive now to return to the model that shows motor and sensory to be inseparable, requiring that visual and motor components be assessed together and addressed as very much interrelated. It is postulated that as inaccurate information is being received from the proprioceptive centers (because of the sensory and motor deficits related to neurological damage), the perception of the body in space will change, and as the perception of the body in space changes, motor components, such as motor control, posture, balance, and coordination will be affected. This interrelationship is important to reinforce, as treating the motor side of the loop will affect visual perception and treating visual perception will affect motor functioning. For example, visual–perceptual neglect, impaired motor function, and decreased sensation in the affected side are frequently noted as simultaneous symptoms that affect one another. It has been the observation of some clinicians that in some cases visual field loss has been partially resolved with the return of other neurological mechanisms, such as motor or sensory (tactile), to reinforce the reinstatement of perception of that visual space, which corresponds motorically (e.g., as sensation and motor return are noted in the left extremities, concurrent opening of the visual field to the left is also noted). This has been an observation only, but serves to reinforce the model of the ambient visual processing system and the sensorimotor feedback loop as a possible or partial explanation for such events.

Hemiplegia and Visual Midline Shift Syndrome

In addition to or in combination with the perceptual deficits just described, a shift in perceptual midline is frequently noted both perceptually and behaviorally in those patients who are post-CVA or head trauma. VMSS (as defined by Padula, 1996) is theorized to be caused by the ambient visual process dysfunction changing orientation to the concept of midline through spatial distortion. Given a neurological event such as a CVA causing hemiparesis or hemiplegia, sensorimotor input from one side of the body is disrupted at the same time that integration of these systems may be disturbed centrally, causing a breakdown in the integration and the accurate perception of the body itself and its location in space.

The ambient process is a relative processing system, and it attempts to create a relative balance on the basis of the information established. Given the interference in the information received from one side of the body relative to the other, the ambient visual process attempts to recreate a spatial relationship that corresponds to the mismatch of information received from the sensorimotor feedback loop. This phenomenon causes a shift in the concept of midline, usually shifting away from the involved side: a midline shift to the right with a left hemiplegia, for example (see Figures 4.3 and 4.4). Midline concepts can shift in the anterior–posterior axis, causing the midline to be shifted forward or backward (see Figures 4.5 and 4.6). When a midline shift exists, the person will relate on testing when a wand or other object is moved across the visual field that the object is in front of his or her nose when it is in fact lateral, above, or below the nose. Combinations of the anterior–posterior and lateral shifts are also common. VMSS fre-

VISUAL MIDLINE SHIFT TEST

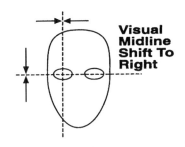

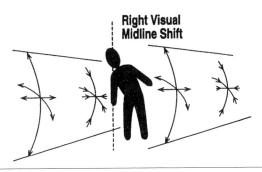

Figure 4.3. Visual midline shift to the right.
From *Neuro-Optometric Rehabilitation.* Copyright © 2000 Optometric Extension Program.
Reprinted with permission.

VISUAL MIDLINE SHIFT TEST

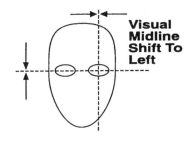

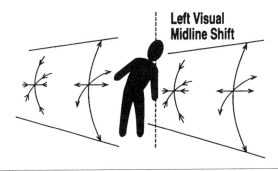

Figure 4.4. Visual midline shift to the left.
From *Neuro-Optometric Rehabilitation.* Copyright © 2000 Optometric Extension Program.
Reprinted with permission.

VISUAL MIDLINE SHIFT TEST

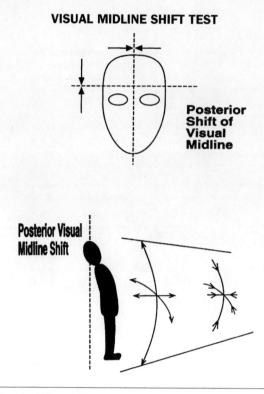

Posterior Shift of Visual Midline

Posterior Visual Midline Shift

Figure 4.5. Posterior visual midline shift.
From *Neuro-Optometric Rehabilitation.* Copyright © 2000 Optometric Extension Program. Reprinted with permission.

quently causes the person to lean toward where midline is perceived to be while resisting weight bearing into the involved or hemiplegic side. The opposite is also noted, though, in behavior that has been termed the *pusher syndrome* by some neurodevelopmental therapists. This behavior entails the person pushing their weight into the hemiplegic, often visually neglected side, while avoiding weight bearing into the uninvolved side. The mechanism for this is not fully understood, but it is the experience of the authors that this behavior is most commonly noted in those with more severe or dense infarcts or bleeds. When a midline shift occurs in the near–far axis, the person will be observed to be leaning into an extensor or flexor pattern while resisting weight shifting in the opposite direction. Any therapist who has experience with this type of case has observed that this resistance to weight bearing can be extreme, as the patients feel they are falling because they perceive the therapist is pushing them way beyond their midline. In the example of a person with a posterior midline shift, leaning forward for a normal sit-to-stand position can be frightening and the person's extensor tone will increase. Another way to understand this concept of the distortion of space through the coupling of an amplification and relative compression of different portions of space is to think of the person's perception as being as if the floor is tilted either laterally, up- or downhill, or a combination. Some people who are cognitively able may say the floor appears tilted. This spatial distortion causes

VISUAL MIDLINE SHIFT TEST

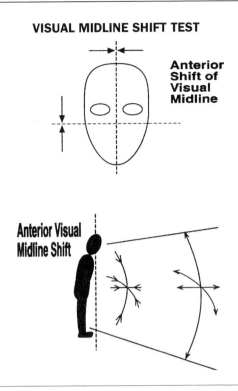

Figure 4.6. Anterior visual midline shift.
From *Neuro-Optometric Rehabilitation.* Copyright © 2000 Optometric Extension Program.
Reprinted with permission.

the corresponding appropriate posture; for example, if one were walking uphill, one would lean forward (see Figures 4.3–4.6).

Yoked Prisms

A neuro-optometric approach that has worked effectively in trials with MSS is the use of yoked prisms placed before both eyes with the base pointing in the same direction. It is important to state here that the traditional use of prisms has been from a sensory or sight-only perspective, which also is beneficial. When used in this manner, the prisms are placed with the base away from the affected hemiplegic side to affect a neglect by moving objects in space toward that side to move the eyes more in the direction of the neglect, attempting to increase awareness of the neglected field.

However, the authors and other clinicians have observed that applying the yoked prisms with the base toward the hemiplegic side (frequently the side the person is leaning away from) is noted to be more consistently effective with VMSS. The theory is that the base of the prisms contracts space on the hemiplegic side so that concept of midline is shifted back to a more normal position. This approach is not used in a compensatory manner, rather in a remedial fashion with a regimen prescribed to be used usually a few hours a day specifically during therapy sessions when motor tasks such as balance, coordination, ambulation, and reaching are being performed. The amount of diopter to be used depends on the severity, established through evaluation trials and with the lowest diopter that is effective. It is important to restate that the prisms are used in conjunction with motor tasks in an attempt to affect motor and functional outcomes. Yoked prisms should be used with the following guidance in mind:

Visual Midline Shift	*Prism Orientation*
Right	Base left
Left	Base right
Anterior	Base down
Posterior	Base up

Other Focuses of Treatment

Areas of potential focus in the rehabilitation of the neurologically impaired patient with corresponding treatment ideas are given. It is important to remember that these ideas need to be used simultaneously or in a graded manner to create treatment activities that promote the individual patient's needs and goals.

Wheelchair Positioning

Wheelchair positioning problems arise not only from muscle weakness and abnormal muscle tone, but also are compounded and accentuated by perceptual deficits. Positioning can frequently be a problem with those at Ranchos Los Amigos Scale 1–3, that is, the stages of coma. In addition to muscle control issues, abnormal muscle tone, especially in the head, neck, and trunk, contributes to the challenge of positioning to prevent contracture and skin breakdown. Optometrically, base-in prism and nasal occlusion may be helpful even at this early stage in reducing high tone. Also, if behaviorally a midline shift is apparent that is causing significant leaning or asymmetrical tone, yoked prisms may reduce leaning behaviors. This also is true for positioning of higher-level patients. The authors have found in cases of severe leaning that may cause a falling or hanging of the affected upper extremity, difficulty in feeding, and orthopedic changes promoting pain, the use of yoked prisms to remediate misperception of the body in space has been quite helpful. In addition to these optometric interventions, multisensory feedback experiences, including moving the patient in many positions, allowing vestibular feedback, and providing weight-bearing experiences through the trunk and extremities, will continue to assist and integrate any changes in spatial perception.

Sitting and Standing Balance and Ambulation

Standard therapeutic approaches to remediating deficits in posture and balance, in addition to improving muscle control and strength, are handling activities that reinforce normalization of tone and righting reactions on which to superimpose functional movement, for example, facilitating equal weight shifting side to side with elongation of the trunk on the weight-bearing side during balance activities. In addition, if balance deficits appear to have a more apparent vestibular component, such as complaints of vertigo, specific vestibular programs with graded movement to desensitize or retrain vestibular mechanisms are implemented. As mentioned previously, PTVS or VMSS from disruption of the ambient visual process often affect perception of the body in space and therefore impede balance, normalized posture, and functional mobility. Therefore, in addition to and in conjunction with the above modalities, use of base-in prism and binasal occlusion may reduce the stress on the ambient system, reducing symptoms and assisting the patient with orientation in space. Also, use of yoked prisms to remediate midline shift can be essential in promoting equalized weight shifting for balance and ambulation. Again, the important behaviors to note that are indicative of a shift in midline are a resistance to weight bearing to one side or the other or shifting weight forward into flexion or backward into extension with potentially increased tone toward the direction of the shift. A commonly observed example among patients with posterior midline shift is a resistance to leaning forward in preparation for sit-to-stand with concurrently increased extensor tone that is aggravated by resistance when the therapist pushes the person forward. The person may resist placing his or her feet flat and will instead push the feet into plantar flexion. All these symptoms make perfect sense when one thinks the floor is tilted downward or downhill. Would you lean forward into a downhill slope? In addition, if that same person were ambulating, he or she would be leaning backward with potentially increased extensor tone. In contrast, with anterior midline shift, the therapist might note a flexed, shuffling gait.

Visual Attention, Pursuits, and Saccades

Visual attentional deficits are sometimes evidenced by such behaviors as distractibility, decreased ability to read without assistive techniques such as the use of a finger to scan the page, decreased ability to read for a length of time, scanning a visual acuity chart, and impaired processing of the visual environment as a whole, especially in crowded or busy places. The important idea to reinforce here is that poor scanning abilities and poor visual attention are not best remediated through oculomotor exercises to start (even functional ones such as graded forms of near reading or scanning tasks), but through integration of the ambient processing system through base-in prism, nasal occlusion, and visual tasks requiring an overlap with the motor systems to integrate spatial–temporal concepts, such as a balance activity at the same time that the patient is requested to touch different objects of focus. The tasks and level of skills required can be modified and graded to fit the specific needs of the patient, as long as they incorporate as many of the following systems as can be tolerated: *visual*, including visual attention, convergence, accommodation, pursuits, and saccades; these are used preferably in *functional* activities incorporating tactile, proprioceptive, kinesthetic, and vestibular components. This provides the basis for many therapy activities, such as graded sports activities (both gross and fine motor), crafts, and ADLs graded or modified to encompass the above. A few specific examples are

- A patient with a dense left neglect should be guided verbally, tactilely, or both to place his or her hand on the sink while brushing the teeth. To visually locate the toothpaste just beyond midline to the left, the patient is instructed to glide his or her hand slowly toward that side of the sink while following the hand with his or her eyes until the tube is located both visually and tactilely. At first, the task should be easy to accomplish, including putting the tube just beyond visual awareness and perhaps giving the patient therapist assistance with a hand-over-hand technique.

- The patient should maintain focus on an object in space that he or she is touching while on a balance board. Focusing on a point in space while ambulating assists the patient in stabilizing peripheral spatial awareness.

- The patient is requested to visually track toward and attend to the cone being manipulated with neurodevelopment theory techniques that incorporate trunk rotation and weight bearing into the affected side in such activities as cone stacking. This needs to be graded in the beginning so the patient can easily access the cone.

Documentation of Services

Information has been presented to provide the therapist with a framework both for complete assessment and remediation of common visual–motor deficits observed in neurologically involved patients. A clear statement of methods used in assessment and treatment will assist in documentation to facilitate reimbursement. Visual-spatial deficits very much impede progress in many potential areas of rehabilitation focus, including but not limited to the following:

- Wheelchair positioning to prevent orthopedic changes, promote posture for ADL such as feeding, and facilitate equal weight bearing for normalized motor return

- Normalizing posture and weight bearing during transfers, standing balance training, and ambulation to promote improved functioning in these areas

- Promoting awareness of the affected extremities to improve the probability of motor return and to promote awareness of body scheme for use in all self-care tasks

- Improving attention to all quadrants of visual space for localizing functional objects in space (including reading and writing)

- Improving overall attention, memory, and cognitive flexibility for improved independence with functional tasks.

The theoretical information in this chapter provides a basis to relate visual–perceptual remedial intervention to these rehabilitation goals and in fact more than implies an incorporation of a visual–perceptual focus into other rehabilitation tasks such as balance, postural work, ADL, and so forth. Each will improve most effectively when combined with the other. Therefore, documentation of rehabilitation time spent in this way can be stated in specific functional terms as part of the treatment plan as any modality such as neuromuscular reeducation is part of a treatment plan to improve transfers, ambulation, and functional motor return.

References

Bandler, R. (1985). *Using your brain for a change.* Moab, UT: Real People Press.

Liebowitz, H. W., & Post, R. B. (1982). The two modes of processing concept and some implications. In J. J. Beck (Ed.), *Organization and representation in perception.* Hillsdale, NJ: Erlbaum.

Nelson, C., & de Benabib, R. (1992). 1992 Conference on Head-Neck Treatment Issues, Cuernavaca, Mexico.

Padula, W. V. (1996). *Neuro-optometric rehabilitation.* Optometric Extension Program Foundation, Inc., 1921 East Carnegie Avenue, Suite 3L, Santa Ana, CA 92705.

Padula, W. V., Argyris, S., & Ray, J. (1994). Visual evoked potentials (VEP) evaluating treatment for post-trauma vision syndrome (PTVS) in patients with traumatic brain injuries (TBI). *Brain Injury, 8,* 125–133.

Trevarthen, C. B., & Sperry, R. W. (1973). Perceptual unity of the ambient visual field in human commissurotomy patients. *Brain,* 564–570.

Wolfe. (1968). *Anatomy of the eye and orbit.* Philadelphia: W. B. Saunders.

Selected Readings

Ayres, A. J. (1973). *Sensory integration and learning disorders.* Los Angeles: Western Psychological Services.

Ayres, A. J. (1979). *Sensory integration and the child.* Los Angeles: Western Psychological Services.

Buktenica, N. (1968). *Visual learning.* Sioux Falls, SD: Adapt Press.

Corbin, C. B. (1980). *A textbook of motor development.* Dubuque, IA: Wm. C. Brown.

Held, R. (1965). Plasticity in sensory–motor systems. *Scientific American, 213,* 84–95.

Ilg, F., & Ames, L. (1995). *Child behavior.* New York: Harper & Row.

Langley, B., & Dubrose, R. (1976). Functional vision screening for severely handicapped children. *New Outlook for Blind, 70,* 346–350.

Trevarthan, C. B., & Speery, R. (1973). Perceptual unity of the ambient visual field in human commissurotomy patients. *Brain, 96,* 547–570.

Driving and Visual Information Processing in Cognitively At-Risk and Older Individuals

Rosamond Gianutsos, PhD, FAAO, CDRS

Although few people question the importance of visual information processing for the safe operation of a motor vehicle, the relationship between vision and driving is surprisingly controversial (Nouri, Tinson, & Lincoln, 1987). Although virtually all states in the United States and most countries have a minimum standard for acuity (often 20/40 or 6/12), researchers and experienced driver rehabilitation specialists (Ramsey, 1990) question the importance of acuity per se, citing examples of people who have driven safely with poor acuity. These experts believe that a much more critical, if not the most critical, factor is the integrity of the visual fields. Their evidence, however, is based largely on clinical experience rather than formal research: A study by Johnson and Keltner (1983) is one of the few available reports. Others (Shinar & Scheiber, 1991) have emphasized the importance of dynamic visual acuity, and still others (Wang, Kosinski, Schwartzbert, & Shanklin, 2003) have emphasized the importance of contrast sensitivity. The controversy sometimes is directed toward emphasizing the relative importance of more cognitive functions, most notably attention (Owsley & Ball, 1993). The relationship between driving and vision becomes significant in individuals who are cognitively at risk, for example, from brain injury or advanced age.

Before examining the specifics of the relationship between vision and driving in cognitively at-risk individuals, it is important to consider some general issues about human abilities and safe driving. Nobody would dispute the fact that driving is an extremely complex form of human behavior for which many competencies are either required or helpful (Colsher & Wallace, 1993; van Zomeren, Brouwer, & Minderhoud,

1987). The American Medical Association has published a significant integration of current thinking about medical conditions and driving (Wang et al., 2003). In this chapter, I summarize state laws, including visual standards, for driving. Although there may not be a consensus regarding what should be required, there is more agreement on what is helpful. For instance, binocular vision is not required for operation of an ordinary motor vehicle; however, it is helpful in that it affords an appreciation of space, especially at night when texture gradient information (an important monocular cue for depth) is lost. Monocular drivers usually develop other techniques for evaluating spatial information.

It is important to note that, when multiple impairments are present, the combined effect may be considerably greater than the sum of the individual parts (Colsher & Wallace, 1993). In research, the components are called *main effects,* and the combined effect is called the *interaction effect.* Impairments of two helpful competencies may produce an interaction (combined effect) that is deadly. For example, my experience with profoundly amnesic survivors of herpes simplex encephalitis—none of whom stopped driving—convinces me that it is possible to drive safely despite extremely poor recent memory; however, such amnesia combined with impulsivity can lead to dangerous lane changes and last-minute turns to cope with a forgotten route. Arthritic changes, common in elderly people, may impede neck rotation and, consequently, over-the-shoulder head checks for traffic in adjacent lanes. These changes could have a particularly serious effect when combined with peripheral field loss associated with glaucoma.

On the other hand, cognitively intact individuals may indeed be able to deal with substantial but isolated and well-recognized impairments. A psychologist (Chapman, 1995) who had been struggling for 25 years with progressive loss of visual acuity due to Stargardt's disease described his own experience driving with field constriction associated with the use of special bioptic (telescope-like) lenses. He drove more than 650,000 miles (~1,050,000 km) with the bioptic lenses and has only recently begun to limit his driving. In his experience, it was only when his acuity worsened to 20/240, correctable to 20/40, and fields narrowed to below 6.5°, that he began to question his ability to drive safely. Most jurisdictions that have standards for visual fields and driving specify well over 100° in the horizontal meridian; it is astounding that this man could drive safely with such narrow fields.

However, it would be a mistake to conclude that peripheral vision is unimportant for driving. The logical error is failing to take into account the interaction effects: The effects of disabilities tend to combine multiplicatively, not additively. Although a well-functioning person might be able to compensate for constriction of the visual fields, with cognitive impairment such compensation may require attention and other mental resources that are unavailable or required for other tasks.

A positive view of interaction effects is to appreciate that there is much to gain from fixing a relatively small impairment that multiplies the impairment caused by another condition. If, for instance, reduced distance visual acuity (a relatively minor impediment to safe driving) is corrected, the benefit may be a disproportionate gain of attentional resources previously needed to compensate for the poor acuity.

Wood (1993) and Szlyk, Brigell, and Seiple (1993) have considered the combined effects on driving of visual and cognitive impairment. Many conditions that cause cognitive impairment also cause visual impairment, so this combination is, unfortunately, not rare. The good news is that many visual problems can be treated, and some can be rectified, without unusual expense, technology, or effort.

What conditions put a driver into the category "cognitively at risk"? Anything that affects the brain can compromise cognitive function. Here, the emphasis is on individuals with an "acquired" brain injury—who developed normally until the onset of some event or condition affected brain function. Usually, such people are seeking to resume or to continue driving. People with developmental disabilities, especially cerebral palsy and spina bifida, present a complex challenge for driver rehabilitation specialists, although this is not addressed in this chapter specifically. Another more common, but less widely recognized, etiology that renders people at risk for unsafe driving is attention deficit disorder, with or without hyperactivity. This condition usually does not combine with physical or visual disability.

The major etiologies to be considered include acquired brain injury (with cerebrovascular accident and traumatic brain injury [TBI] being the most common) and age-associated cognitive decline. People with progressive neurological conditions, such as multiple sclerosis, Alzheimer's disease, and other forms of dementia, present similar issues, together with some specialized considerations (e.g., the visual problems specific to multiple sclerosis) that are beyond the scope of this chapter. In cases in which progression, variability in symptom expression, or recurrence is anticipated, there must be guidelines for reevaluating a person's driving risk. Initial evaluation done early in the disease process can be used to establish a personal baseline and triggers for reviewing the situation. Planning can be started for mobility alternatives.

Age-associated cognitive impairment, although not universal, and sometimes caused by correctable but undiagnosed problems, is a reality, especially as advances in medical treatment keep people living longer, and in better physical health. In some sense, the issues are similar to progressive conditions.

Stroke is the most common form of acquired brain injury, with older people at increased risk. The most likely physical impairment following stroke is hemiplegia. The most common visual problem is hemifield impairment, with or without hemi-inattention. TBI often strikes younger, and sometimes, inexperienced, risk-prone drivers. Physical impairment, although similar to stroke, can be more severe, especially following a prolonged loss of consciousness and immobility. Problems with motor coordination, balance, and vestibular function are not unusual after brain trauma. Not only may there be visual hemifield impairment, but there also is a high incidence of accommodative and binocular dysfunction.

Driver Rehabilitation

Driver rehabilitation has advanced considerably in the past 10 years, especially under the auspices of the Association for Driver Rehabilitation Specialists (formerly the Association of Driver Educators for the Disabled), an interdisciplinary organization of occupational therapists, driver educators, and others. This organization has established a certification process leading to the title *Certified Driver Rehabilitation Specialist*. Adaptation to accommodate physical disabilities is an important part of this specialty, but addressing cognitive and sensory impairment is often a greater challenge. This type of consultation may be called *driving advisement* or *driver consultation*. It includes evaluation, counseling, and intervention.

The essential purpose of driving advisement is to enable the individual to make appropriate decisions about driving. Regardless of the legal context (i.e., some jurisdictions have mandatory reporting by professionals of drivers with certain diagnoses), the would-be driver is the ultimate licensor. On every trip, an implicit self-authorization is given; conversely, from time to time, most drivers make conscious decisions to refrain from driving or to allow others to drive. These decisions are usually to accommodate some fairly obvious condition, such as fatigue, intoxication, or a broken bone. In the domain of vision, glare is a condition that is usually obvious to the driver, and steps are taken either to correct or to avoid it. Older drivers frequently refrain from driving at night because they are sensitive to glare.

Automotive researchers (e.g., Bullough, Fu, & van Derlofske, 2002) have paid much attention to the problem of glare because it has direct bearing on headlamp design, and they have found it necessary to distinguish *disability glare* from *discomfort glare*. The blue-tinged halogen headlamps on newer cars afford increased illumination for the driver; however, drivers of other vehicles complain of glare. It turns out that there is an imperfect relationship: Discomfort with glare is not perfectly correlated with the extent to which glare is disabling. The blue-tinged halogen headlamps may produce discomfort glare but not disability glare. Notwithstanding these distinctions, the bottom line is that little assessment is needed when drivers recognize the problem and perceive it as interfering with their ability to drive safely.

In the assessment part of driving advisement, the priority has to be on those conditions for which awareness may be compromised. A recent study (West et al., 2003) on vision and driving self-restriction in older adults found that, whereas older people with poor depth perception would restrict their driving, those with impairments in the attentional field would not. Awareness is often compromised with visual field impairment. Clinicians will frequently encounter people who have dramatically constricted fields who insist that they are "seeing everything." Hemianopic field losses are typically unappreciated or underappreciated. The most convincing illustration of this phenomenon for a neurologically intact individual is a demonstration in which an object is made to disappear in the area subtended by the physiological blind spot (see Figure 5.1).

L   R

Blind Spot Demonstration

1. Hold at arm's length.
2. Close your left eye and
3. Look at the L with your right eye.
4. Slowly bring the sheet toward you.
5. Keep looking at the L, but notice what happens to the R.
6. At some point you will realize that the R is no longer visible.
7. Keep moving the paper closer and the R will reappear.
8. Repeat the process with the other eye.

Note. Although the letter disappears, the paper does not. This phenomenon is known as the *completion effect.* **The brain fills in gaps in the visual field with predictable patterns or surfaces.**

Figure 5.1. Blind spot demonstration.

Sensory impairment needs to be evaluated because, unlike motor impairment, it can be inferred only indirectly from behavior, and often the impairment does not lend itself to self-evaluation. It seems that the human organism is not built to monitor some sensory functions well. For instance, people with hearing problems may think others are mumbling. Another example is the loss of spatial vision following binocular dysfunction. It is not uncommon for people with dramatic losses of acuity to present themselves for an eye examination with little or no complaint.

The driving advisement process usually includes an in-clinic component and an on-the-road, behind-the-wheel component, typically (for obvious safety reasons), in that order. On occasion, the on-the-road component will be deferred on the basis of severely deficient performance on the in-clinic component. Sometimes, a condition will be identified on the in-clinic component that disqualifies the person from licensure, such as homonymous hemianopia caused by postchiasmic damage in the brain's visual pathways. Terry Grismer successfully challenged the automatic disqualification from driving based on homonymous hemianopia by the British Columbia Superintendent of Motor Vehicles, claiming instead that the state had to prove a functional impairment in driving (*British Columbia [Superintendent of Motor Vehicles] v. British Columbia [Council of Human Rights]*, 1999). A committee on which I served, which was charged with making recommendations regarding what should be included in driver rehabilitation assessment, concluded that no one should be recommended for driving without first demonstrating satisfactory performance on the road (Subcommittee on Driver Evaluation and Training for Individuals with Disabilities, 1993). Some functionally oriented driver rehabilitation specialists discount or minimize the in-clinic findings, placing total reliance on the outcome of the road test. This position may be ill advised, given the limitations of road tests—a subject that is addressed after the in-clinic assessment.

The in-clinic assessment needs to address medical, sensory, motor, and cognitive functions. The medical consideration is the presence of conditions that could produce a rapid change in the person's abilities, including consciousness, vision, debilitating pain, or loss of contact with reality. Included here is the effect of substances, prescribed and otherwise, that might affect the individual's performance. The sensory assessment emphasizes vision—detailed later in this chapter—although joint and position sense are important, especially for reliable and efficient pedal control. Motor function is particularly important in relation to the need for adaptive equipment, including mirrors.

In a clinical regard, I am struck by motor planning problems (dyspraxia) among elderly people. These problems may be an early indicator of dementia and could cause the tragic wrong-pedal crashes that periodically hit the front pages. George Russell Weller, the 86-year-old man who drove through barriers set up for a farmer's market in Santa Monica, California, maintained that he had mistaken the gas pedal for the brake (CNN, Sunday, July 20, 2003). The market obstructed his usual route home. Weller told the police that he did not realize until too late that the avenue was closed to traffic.

I would note that Weller's mistake was not simply hitting the wrong pedal but the inability to make an immediate correction. One of my patients was dragged 40 ft (12 m) by a 78-year-old woman who was making a U-turn close to home. Afterward, the woman said she thought there was something wrong with the car. No defects were found. On the Elemental Driving Simulator (EDS), I commonly observe older people becoming rattled and rushing to make a corrective action that is the opposite of what is needed. Some of them persevere in this action, not only making the wrong decision but also making a bad situation worse by perseveration.

In my opinion, it is in the areas of cognition and vision that the in-clinic assessment can have unique value because in these domains there are hidden problems that may not be safely or intentionally tested on an ordinary road test. I discuss recommendations for the vision screening later. The features of procedures for evaluating cognition in relationship to driving are summarized in Table 5.1.

The critical features include (a) apparent (face) validity, (b) psychometric properties (demonstrated standardization, reliability, and validity), and (c) clinical practicality. Apparent, or face, validity is important if the examinee is to be convinced of the relevance of the findings. It is central to the driving advisement process and must not be discounted as "mere cosmesis." The appeal of the on-road assessment is in its face validity. Simulation attempts to maximize face validity, although procedures vary in what is simulated, ranging from hardware simulations (e.g., the Doron Simulator) to task simulations (e.g., the EDS).

The driving advisement procedures vary in their scope. For example, none, other than the on-road test, addresses binocular depth perception in driving. They also vary in whether they include a defined assessment protocol. Some (e.g., Doron Simulator, neuropsychological assessment) consist of a large collection of potentially useful scenarios or tasks. With regard to psychometric development, it is amazing how often this crucial ingredient has been lacking. The Porto–Clinic Glare—at one time the most widely used evaluation protocol—has norms from 18- and 19-year-old Marine recruits—a fact that was not generally known. No reliability and validity data were offered. Clinical practicality starts with cost of materials but also includes space and therapist time.

Because most existing procedures did not possess all these features, in the late 1980s I developed the Driving Advisement System (Gianutsos, 1988; Gianutsos, Campbell, Beattie, & Mandriota, 1992) and, subsequently, the EDS (Gianutsos, 1994; Gianutsos & Beattie, 1992). Research on the validity of the EDS is summarized in the manual (http://www.cogrehab.com/resources/DRMAN.pdf) and includes significant correlations with an independent on-road assessment (A. Campbell, personal communication, June 21, 1995), at-fault crashes (Brown, Greaney, Mitchel, & Lee, 1993), and limitation of driving by older drivers (DeLibero, 1995). In DeLibero's (1995) study, a group of community-residing older drivers (free of neurological diagnoses) were compared with a young adult group of drivers. EDS performance correlated strongly ($r = .68$) with report-

Table 5.1. Features of Procedures Used for Pre-Driving Advisement: Comparative Summary of Major Driving Assessments

Issue	Porto–Clinic Glare	Driver Performance Test	Doron Simulator	Driving Advisement System	Elemental Driving Simulator	Neuro-psychiatric Testing	On-road Testing	Cognitive Behavioral Driver's Inventory	Visual Attention Analyzer–Useful Field of View	Atari
Face validity	Moderately low	Moderately high	High	Moderately high	Moderately high	Low	Highest	Moderately low	Moderately low	Moderately high
Scope	Focused	Focused	Focused	Broad	Broad	Test dependent	Broad	Broad	Focused	Unknown
Protocol	Standard	Standard	Select procedure	Standard	Standard	Select procedure	No standard	Standard	Standard	No standard
Norms	Marines	Yes	Nonempirical	Yes	Yes	Usually	Rarely	Yes	Yes	No
Reliability	Not reported	Not reported	Not reported	Yes	Yes	Usually	Rarely	Yes	Yes	No
Validity	Not reported	Not reported	Not reported	Yes	Yes	Not for driving	Unknown	Yes	Yes	No
Time (min)	15	45	60+	60+	30	15–60	60	60	Approximately 30	60
Space/equipment (in.)	Tabletop + 20 VCR		Room	Computer	Computer	Tests	Vehicle+	Computer + Test	Console	Console
Cost (estimated)	$1,200	$200	$30,000	$3,500+	$3,500+	< $500	Direct + independent	$120[a]	$20,000	$15,000
Source	DTE[b]	ADSI[c]	Doron[d]	LSA[e]	LSA[e]	Test	Self	PSS[f]	VRI[g]	Atari[h]

[a] Cognitive Behavioral Driver's Inventory requires acquisition of additional test components.
[b] DTE = Driver Testing Equipment, Inc., 1020 S. Main Avenue, Scranton, PA 18504, (717) 347-7772.
[c] ADSI = Advanced Driving Skills Institute, 427 N. Primrose Drive, Orlando, FL 32803.
[d] Doron = Doron Precision Systems, P.O. Box 400, Binghamton, NY 13902, (607) 772-1610.
[e] LSA = Life Science Associates, 1 Fenimore Road, Bayport, NY 11705, (631) 472-2111.
[f] PSS = Psychological Software Services, 6555 Carrollton Avenue, Indianapolis, IN 46220, (317) 257-9672.
[g] VRI = Visual Resources, Inc., 216 S. Jefferson, Suite 600, Chicago, IL 60661, (312) 454-0603.
[h] Atari = Atari Games Corp., 675 Sycamore Drive, Milpitas, CA 95035.

ed driving pattern; specifically, the older drivers not only struggled with the EDS but also reported that they limited their driving (e.g., avoided driving in bad weather, at night, over long distances, and in congested or unfamiliar places). Interestingly enough, these drivers felt they were still above average in their basic abilities! In general, their self-appraisals bore no relationship with their performance; however, it appears that they were making appropriate decisions about driving.

The EDS, which is illustrated in Figure 5.2, is a physically rudimentary simulator. The EDS protocol is designed to address simple and complex reaction time, impulse control, response consistency, lateral responsivity, and steering steadiness. Individuals are asked to predict how well they will do compared with other licensed drivers and are later given norm-referenced performance ratings. Because the predictions and performance are anchored to the same numeric scale, the report affords a direct comparison of the two. If there is a high disparity, indicating that the person has unrealistic expectations, the clinician has a good foundation to address issues of judgment and driving beyond one's capabilities.

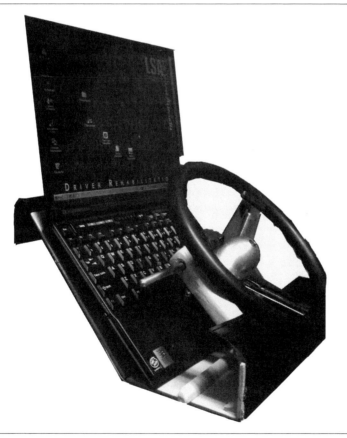

Figure 5.2. The Elemental Driving Simulator, including a laptop computer, steering wheel, and turn signal. A three-pedal assembly (not shown) is placed on the floor and permits analysis of foot pedal control and efficiency.

Licensed drivers who were tested for the purpose of collecting normative information performed consistently and efficiently on the EDS, whereas people who are cognitively at risk often find it quite difficult. Indeed, most feedback is to the effect that the EDS is more difficult than ordinary driving—which is as it should be. Most of the time, driving calls for relaxed vigilance. However, in a heartbeat the task can require complex decisions implemented with precise and rapid timing. What is called for in driving advisement is an aggressive and challenging exploration of all the potential areas of difficulty. It is far better to err in the direction of making the assessment too difficult than too easy.

Performance on the road test is often regarded as the ultimate hurdle, much as it is in the licensure process. Notwithstanding its indisputable face validity, the road tests used in most rehabilitation contexts fail to meet psychometric standards, including reliability and validity. Because driving environments vary, the course varies, as does the behavior of other drivers. Standardization of procedure, and especially of scoring, is therefore difficult to achieve in the usual sense. Reliability and validity are consequently undetermined. Most on-road assessment protocols, based on my own informal survey, emphasize the operational level of driving: the basic skills needed for keeping the vehicle on the road. Little attention is paid to the more proactive tactical (van Zomeren et al., 1987) level of driving, including, for example, route selection, anticipation of erratic behavior based on clues such as out-of-state plates, and deciding whether and when to make a trip. This tactical level of driving calls for just the kind of frontal abilities that are often compromised by TBI. Typically, the road test evaluator assumes full responsibility for the route, which may or may not be a familiar driving environment for the examinee. Similarly, it is often impractical to evaluate performance at different times of day and in different weather conditions.

The evaluation process is an evolving clinical art and far from perfect. Important as the on-road test is, especially to the would-be driver, it should not be the only or ultimate test. If a person does poorly on the in-clinic procedures but does well on the on-road test, it does not mean that the in-clinic procedures should be discounted or overridden (trumped) by the road test findings. The ultimate successful outcome is the accumulation of safe miles.

Visual Processing and Impact on Driving

Based on years of clinical experience, in a masterful application of an understanding of basic processes to an important activity of daily living, occupational therapist Carmella Strano analyzed the specific visual problems associated with brain injury and their impact on specific aspects of the driving task (Strano, 1989). Complementing Strano's analysis is Shinar and Scheiber's (1991) review of empirical research on this topic.

In clinical practice, static acuity is addressed first and, as mentioned earlier, static distance acuity is almost universally included in licensure standards, but it is thought to be overemphasized. However, it can be important in unfamiliar situations in which information must be derived from signs. Good distant acuity can allow for earlier recognition of potential hazards, such as where the other driver is looking.

Contrast sensitivity, often reduced in older people, can affect safety in night driving and in conditions where visibility is compromised by bad weather (Schiff, Arnone, & Cross, 1994). It is one of the most consistent correlates of ultimate driving safety. Practical contrast sensitivity materials have become available for therapists, including the Vistech wall chart; the Pelli–Robson chart; contrast sensitivity plates in stereoscopic vision screeners; and comparative high- and low-contrast acuity charts, such as are included in the AARP publication "Older Driver Skill Assessment and Resource Guide: Creating Mobility Choices" (Stock No. D14957, AARP Fulfillment, P.O. Box 96796, Washington, DC 20090-6796).

Some investigators (Shinar & Scheiber, 1991) have emphasized the importance for driving of *dynamic acuity*—the ability to discriminate information in moving stimuli. Dynamic acuity is most likely mediated by different neurological systems for vision and receptors for motion as opposed to light intensity, for example, what Suter (1995) called the *magnocellular* or "where" pathway, together with a midbrain "ambient" system. In a clinical sense, the distinction between conventional static and dynamic acuity has helped explain the mobility of some people with apparently poor vision. Unfortunately, clinically practical methods for evaluating dynamic acuity remain unavailable.

Format (iconic vs. verbal); size of letters; and the width, color, and composition of roadway markings are all parameters that can be used by highway planners and engineers to overcome problems with acuity. Individuals can often make changes in the routes they drive, even though they are usually unable to change the roadways. A personally unforgettable exception is my own father, who sought my assistance in finding a good source of reflectors. Later, I discovered that he had installed them at a difficult, otherwise-unmarked turn!

Near-point acuity is unlikely to be important for most aspects of driving, other than to read maps and certain gauges on the dashboard. Car manufacturers are increasing the contrast and size of displays to minimize the impact of reduced near-point acuity, presumably in anticipation of an increasing market of senior drivers with presbyopia and macular degeneration.

The dynamic functions of the visual system—those that depend on coordinated use of the musculature in the eyes—support binocularity, accommodation, and eye movements. Each can be helpful to the driver. For example, stereopsis (a product of binocular function) affords a three-dimensional appreciation of space. Loss of binocular function, and hence stereopsis, is common after TBI. If a person uses an eye patch to manage diplopia, or has lost an eye, stereopsis is lost. Less well appreciated, but possibly more frequent, is the loss of stereopsis in early stages of conditions that affect elderly people (e.g., cataracts, macular degeneration) in which one eye is impaired first. The driver can use stereopsis in parking and making judgments about following distance and gaps in the traffic flow for merges and turns. Stopping too soon or too late at intersections is a symptom of poor stereopsis.

It is important to recognize that there is a fairly high incidence of impaired stereopsis in the general population and that a patient may never have had stereopsis. History is the best way to evaluate this possibility: People in certain occupations—for example, pilots, police officers, and commercial truck drivers—are required to have binocular vision and probably have had stereopsis. On the other hand, people who may never have had stereopsis are those who had an eye turn when young or were given patching or eye exercises in childhood. Under these circumstances, there was nothing to lose, and in all likelihood the person can still use the monocular spatial analysis cues used before the injury. Bear in mind that it is the *loss* of stereopsis, not simply the *lack* of stereopsis, which is significant for driver rehabilitation. Other than for commercial drivers (who require binocular vision for licensure), this loss can usually be addressed through patient education and supervised practice. Optometric evaluation and vision therapy treatment should be considered, as these interventions may enhance the individual's quality of life as well as his or her ability to drive safely.

Eye movement disorders, especially those characterized by spontaneous eye movements (nystagmus), are often difficult to treat. Under these circumstances, acuity is likely to be reduced and should be checked carefully. Glasses will not correct acuity loss caused by nystagmus. If there is a restricted range of eye movement, mirrors and explicit head turns may enable safe driving.

Accommodative function may be helpful in allowing the driver to adjust his or her focus from road to console. To address the loss of accommodation that is almost universal in older drivers, automotive engineers have designed "Heads up" displays in which important dashboard information appears projected into space on or in front of the windshield. Because the information is designed to appear farther away, it is an advantage to older drivers who have lost the ability to adjust focus easily from far to near point. Bi-, multi-, or variable-focus lenses also help compensate for loss of accommodation. In most cases, this problem is easily and routinely addressed.

At the opposite end of the spectrum, neither easily nor routinely addressed, are visual field impairments. These have been alluded to throughout, and readers are referred to other works by myself and others on the subject (Gianutsos & Suchoff, 1996; Parisi, Bell, & Yassein, 1991). Visual field loss is compounded by a total or partial lack of awareness. If homonymous hemianopia (loss of visual responsivity in corresponding halves of the field of view) were experienced as a black stage curtain covering the field, it is unlikely that the individual would consider driving.

When hemianopics attempt to drive, or perform dynamic visual search tasks, they often display a "robbing Peter to pay Paul" effect. They are so busy compensating that they fail to notice something on the intact side. This effect is also seen in steering, in that they have difficulty maintaining a central position in their lane. At times, they may drift too far into their missing field; at other times, they drift into the intact field.

Because visual field impairment disqualifies one for licensure in many jurisdictions and is regarded by many as incompatible with safe driving, there is little opportunity to evaluate whether it can be done. For that reason it is perhaps appropriate to share my own clinical experiences in this regard. The EDS affords an extremely sensitive measure of responsivity to peripheral stimuli on the left and right sides while performing a preview tracking (steering) task. In 95% of the normative sample, the difference in median response time is less than 0.10 s. If a person is 0.5 s slower on one side, the result will be flagged as extremely abnormal. Nonetheless, in more than one such case driving performance was acceptable to an experienced road test examiner instructed to address this potential problem rigorously. Another individual with a dense left homonymous hemianopia from a stroke 6 months earlier continued to drive against advice. He bumped into furniture in the examiner's office, got lost, and could not fill out a paper-and-pencil form. On the EDS, he was 1.5 s slower on the left side, and he missed some targets altogether. Nevertheless, he did well on other assessments, was well aware of the visual loss, and explicitly attempted to compensate. He insisted on continuing to drive. In New York State, his field loss would have come to the attention of the licensing authorities only if his best corrected visual acuity were marginal, and he would have been required to submit a visual evaluation report. New York State does not afford immunity to concerned professionals for reporting such cases. Under the circumstances, I reluctantly urged him to pursue optical compensation using a reversing spectacle mounted mirror, and eventually he did so.

I am aware of at least three cases in which people with right homonymous hemianopia have driven for several years, one with a reversing mirror. Two eventually stopped driving. In each case, the final mishap was a crash in which the field problem was likely to have been contributory, although in neither case did this information come to the attention of the authorities. For instance, shortly after turning left onto a busy two-way commercial street, one of these individuals hit a parked bakery delivery van on his right side.

One young man, whose head trauma left him with a dense right homonymous hemianopia, shown in the lower panel of Figure 5.3, continues to drive safely and without significant restriction. Although he struggles with short-term memory problems, he has been able to maintain employment, albeit at a level below what would be expected on the basis of his training. Most significant, in my opinion, is his ability to describe and depict his visual field loss, as shown in the subjective visual field drawings in the upper panel of Figure 5.3. This degree of awareness is unusual for people with visual field losses.

Another person, a survivor of a severe stroke that left him with profound expressive aphasia, right hemiplegia, and a reduced visual responsivity in the lower right quadrant, amassed over 100,000 safe miles (~161,000 km). He actively denied any visual field

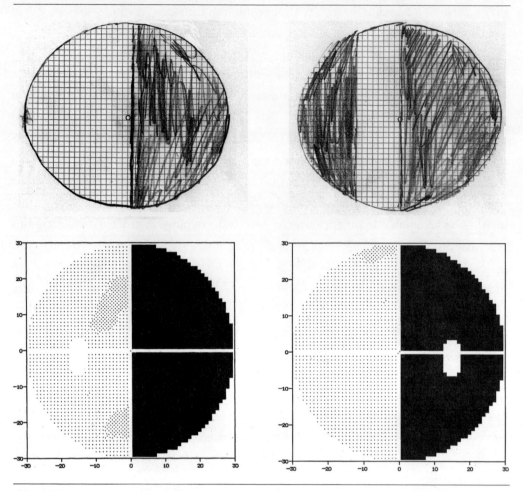

Figure 5.3. Subjective (upper panel) and perimetric (lower panel) visual fields for a right homonymous hemianopic head trauma survivor who successfully resumed driving.

impairment, although there were consistent reductions in response on functional visual field tasks (Gianutsos, 1991). However, for a month or two during which he was given a medication that made him drowsy, he had three minor scrapes on his right side. After stopping the medication, he once again drove safely.

My opinion is that it is very difficult for a person with homonymous hemianopia to maintain a safe driving record. In some cases, where the problem is isolated and awareness is good, it may be possible to drive safely with mirrors and optical aids, for example, oversized, wide-angle, center-mounted rear-view mirrors; reversing mirrors; and yoked prisms (Cohen & Waiss, 1993). Furthermore, the amount and kind of driving may make a difference. Optometrist Daniel Gottlieb has reported favorably on this approach (Gottlieb, 1993; Gottlieb, Freeman, & Williams, 1992).

My own rehabilitative approach is to demonstrate the problem to the patient by offering speeded visual processing tasks in which there is feedback based on stimulus position. If the person can compensate on one task, switch to another. Let the person attempt to generalize compensation to the new task. Increase the information density (visual complexity) of the display or the task complexity. Does the problem reemerge when the task is difficult, or when the individual is tired? Have the person analyze and tabulate his or her performance, broken down by side of display. If the person does well on these off-road tasks and qualifies for driving lessons, be sure the driving instructor observes carefully for problems symptomatic of lateralized differential response and brings them quickly and bluntly to the individual's attention. Even with an optical device, the driver with hemianopsis must maintain an extraordinary level of vigilance. Such drivers should be monitored over an extended period; encouraged to keep a driving log; and to discuss their experiences, including near misses.

Visual attention and visual perception have a significant cognitive aspect; however, they are built on a foundation of visual sensory processing, which, logically and practically, should be addressed first. The practical reason is that visual sensory function can often be treated, if not fixed, more easily than attention and perception can. Instead of *attention*, it would be preferable to use terms that differentiate the aspects of information processing, including the following six phrases: (a) *arousal*, (b) *sustaining a focus of effort*, (c) *resisting distraction*, (d) *selecting relevant and filtering out irrelevant information*, (e) *simultaneous or divided information processing*, and (f) *mental flexibility* or *switching from one level or aspect to another efficiently*. Because of these many different meanings, *attention* (together with *motivation*) is often used as a scapegoat or "explanation" for variability that is not understood (in which case it is an instance of the nominal fallacy; naming something is not explaining it). A person responds inconsistently to stimuli presented to the field of vision contralateral to his or her brain injury: it is explained as "hemi-inattention." A boy is erratic about completing his schoolwork: His "motivation" is questioned, or he may be suspected of having attention deficit disorder.

With that caveat in mind, there are very real attentional problems associated with cognitive impairment that profoundly affect driving (Brouwer, Waterink, van Wolffelaar, & Rothengatter, 1991; Parasuraman & Nestor, 1993). It is possible to identify specific aspects of driving that require each of the six types of attention cited above (Mitchell, 1994). The best clinical research on this subject addresses the constriction in the *useful field of view* (UFOV) among older drivers (Ball & Owsley, 1991; Owsley & Ball, 1993; Owsley, Ball, Sloane, Roenker, & Bruni, 1991). Owsley, Ball, and their collaborators have demonstrated that recent driving records correlate with UFOV performance, that UFOV can predict driving, and that training can be used to counter these effects. The UFOV is a field of visual attention. One way to understand it is to consider the constriction of awareness that people experience when they are working hard on a specific task, such as being engrossed in a book or a movie. UFOV research has been used to account for the fact that older drivers have a disproportionate number of crashes making left turns at intersections, for which they need to deal with multiple issues in real time, such as judging the gap in oncoming traffic, monitoring pedestrians, being aware of other drivers who may also be turning, and controlling their vehicle.

The field of visual attention can be assessed in several ways. A straightforward approach is to evaluate the functional visual fields using increasingly complex displays. Although all people need more time to process informationally dense displays, some are more affected by the increase in information density than others. Using this approach, detailed elsewhere (Gianutsos, 1996; Gianutsos & Suchoff, 1996), one can differentiate the contribution of sensory and attentional field impairment. Older drivers have more difficulty, relative to younger drivers, on the informationally complex tasks (Hall, 1995).

Finally, visual perception includes the interpretation of visual information. Recognition of objects (*visual gnosis*) may be delayed or impaired altogether. Knowing that something constitutes a hazard is critical to dealing with it appropriately. The old saw that a driver "must expect the unexpected" is an implicit acknowledgment of the importance of efficient visual perception in driving. Visual perception is clearly important in finding one's way (route finding).

Vision Screening for Driving

What, then, is recommended as a visual screening procedure in conjunction with driving advisement? With candidates for driving advisement, a stereoscopic vision test can efficiently assess most of the aspects of vision cited earlier as particularly relevant for driving: acuity, binocular function, and horizontal visual field. However, it is no longer acceptable for therapists to use this type of procedure as a substitute for a comprehensive examination by an eye care practitioner (an optometrist or ophthalmologist.) Vision screenings do not identify medical conditions such as glaucoma and cataracts; neither are they adequate for the identification and management of binocular system disorders. On the other hand, it is still not uncommon for ophthalmologic examinations to overlook binocularity and oculomotor functions. A therapist who suspects that binocularity has not been addressed in an eye examination might pursue it with a stereoscopic screening test or a booklet screening for stereopsis (e.g., Randot, StereoFly. Both of these are supplied by Stereo Optical, Inc., 3539 N. Kenton Ave., Chicago, IL 60641; http://www.stereooptical.com/MainPages/Randot.htm). Positive findings would then help justify referral to an eye care practitioner (usually an optometrist) who will address the matter.

More and more frequently, eye doctors are including automated perimetric visual field testing as part of their evaluations. It is often described to patients as the "side vision test." In one recent case, an older woman produced a visual field report that showed an almost 75% loss in corresponding areas of both eyes. This test had been conducted 18 months earlier, during which time she had continued to drive. Clinical assessment indicated that the problem had not resolved. She had had one crash in which her pattern of field loss was a likely contributing factor. We will never know whether her eye doctor advised her not to drive but what we do know is that she and her family had no idea of the extent of her loss.

Overall, occupational therapists should address their efforts toward bringing about an appropriate and comprehensive eye examination and assisting in appropriate understanding of, and follow through on, recommendations. Usually, the eye care practitioner will appreciate the therapist's help in working with patients who have known or suspected cognitive problems.

An area that therapists should explore thoroughly is the functional visual field, particularly for the periphery. I use a collection of computerized tasks (Reaction Time Measure of Visual Field [REACT], the Single and Double Simultaneous Stimulation Test [SDSST], Search for the Odd Shape, and Searching for Shapes) in which the attentional demands are progressively increased. These tasks (Gianutsos & Suchoff, 1996), which are together called PERFIELD, are very practical in that they may be conducted with most IBM-compatible computers. Normative data for younger and older adults accompany the programs. A summary sheet (Exhibit 5.1) is useful to guide this part of the evaluation.

The REACT task is always used first. The task, which takes about 2.5 min, is repeated several times, with varying conditions. It is initially conducted binocularly, with the eyes free to move, and normal contrast. The examiner encourages response speed, especially on the central trials, which come first. Attention is drawn to the fact that the numbers that appear measure reaction time and that the goal is to get as low a score as possible. To explore the effect of distraction, the examiner can tell the patient "We need to do this again, but you can answer some questions for me." Similarly, one can investigate the effects of fixation versus having the eyes free to move and the effects of high and low contrast. The latter is most conveniently accomplished by testing the individual with special dark glasses that filter all but 1% of the light, that is, 1% transmission gray–green wrap-around lenses (very dark sunglasses) for implementing REACT low-contrast conditions. (These are available from NoIR Medical Technologies, P.O. Box 159, South Lyon, MI 48178; 800-521-9746.) These can be placed over existing glasses, and the patient often interprets the procedure as addressing night driving, although no claims are made in that regard. The REACT task conducted monocularly with fixation is most comparable to perimetric visual field testing. With his or her eyes free to move, the individual is given the opportunity to demonstrate compensation for field loss. When hemianopic impairment is observed only with dark glasses, it is likely that there is a relative, but not absolute, loss.

The SDSST is a computerized version of the Single and Double Simultaneous Stimulation Test, where stimuli are flashed on one or both sides in discrete trials. The computer tabulates omissions and confusions by side of the display for single and double presentations. The classic "extinction" pattern, which is actually rather rare, is for errors on the affected side to occur only on double trials.

The Search for the Odd Shape task involves the scanning of an array of shapes ("Martian faces") for one that is different, for example, the Martian that "fell asleep", and

Exhibit 5.1. Form for Organizing Data From Functional Visual Field Tasks

Peripheral Visual Field: Functional Assessment

Patient: _____ ID# _____

Examiner: _____

Date: _____

Procedures: _____

REACT (Reaction Time Measure of Visual Field)

	Eye Tested	Fixate /Move	Dynamic /Stable	Contrast	Dis- traction	Mean Left	Mean Center	Mean Right	Median Left	Median Center	Median Right	Comment
1.	OU	M	D	full	N	___	___	___	___	___	___	___
2.	OU	M	D	full	Y	___	___	___	___	___	___	___
3.	OD	F	D	full	N	___	___	___	___	___	___	___
4.	OS	F	D	full	N	___	___	___	___	___	___	___
5.	OD	F	D	1%	N	___	___	___	___	___	___	___
6.	OS	F	D	1%	N	___	___	___	___	___	___	___
7.	___	___	S	___	___	___	___	___	___	___	___	___
8.	___	___	___	___	___	___	___	___	___	___	___	___
9.	___	___	___	___	___	___	___	___	___	___	___	___
10.	___	___	___	___	___	___	___	___	___	___	___	___

Variables addressed:

__ Eyes free to move vs. eyes fixated

__ Binocular / monocular

__ Normal vs. reduced contrast

__ Without vs. with distraction

__ Dynamic / stable

Interpretation:

Field problems?:

Compensation?:

Prismatic assist: Effect:

SDSST (Single and Double Simultaneous Stimulation)

Administration   1: _____   2: _____

Overall correct / N of trials: _____ / _____   _____ / _____

Errors

		Left	Right	Left	Right	Pattern of impairment:
Single	Confusions	___	___	___	___	
	Omissions	___	___	___	___	Left or right side
	Intrusions	___	___	___	___	Confusion vs. omission
Double	Confusions	___	___	___	___	'Extinction' (Double << Single)
	Omissions	___	___	___	___	Prismatic assist: Effect:

Visual Search — SOSH (Search for the Odd Shape) and SEARCH for shapes

Search Times

	Left	Right	Both
SOSH			
Median	___	___	___
Mean	___	___	___
SEARCH			
Median	___	___	___
Mean	___	___	___
Error %	___	___	___

Interpretation:

poking him to "wake him up," the faster the better. This task is easy to understand and perform; however, some peoples who have sustained brain injuries first begin to encounter difficulty on this task. This pattern suggests reduced attentional capacity. This effect may be even more pronounced on the Searching for Shapes task. On both tasks, the search times are displayed in the target location and summarized by quadrant and side.

One helpful feature of the PERFIELD procedures is that the results are displayed immediately in a format that the patient can understand. This feedback is of special value because it helps the individual become aware of visual field impairment.

Perceptual problems can be investigated using a road sign recognition task. Striking perceptual problems are often revealed in people with dementia. A formalized version of this procedure, with scoring guidelines and normative data, is needed. In the meantime, one can create an assessment by scanning road signs from the Department of Motor Vehicles student manual and removing the labels.

Conclusion

These procedures clearly go well beyond the minimal standards for licensure. After all, driving advisement is for the purpose of giving the individual all the relevant information. Although addressing the issue of whether the person meets the minimal standards for licensure is appropriate, it is not sufficient. The decision is the responsibility of the licensing authorities and, in a deeper sense, which I discussed at the beginning of this chapter, the prospective driver and concerned others. In driver rehabilitation, the therapist is charged with identifying problems in functions that ordinarily are helpful for safe driving. In weighing the information and formulating recommendations, one must keep in mind the potential for compounding of impairments (interaction effects).

References

Ball, K., & Owsley, C. (1991). Identifying correlates of accident involvement for the older driver. *Human Factors, 33,* 583–595.

British Columbia (Superintendent of Motor Vehicles) v. British Columbia (Council of Human Rights) (1999), 36 C.H.R.R. D/129 (S.C.C.); rev'g (1997), 30 C.H.R.R. D/446 (B.C.C.A.); rev'g (1996), 25 C.H.R.R. D/309 (B.C.S.C.); aff'g (sub nom. Grismer v. British Columbia (Attorney General)) (1994), 25 C.H.R.R. D/296 (B.C.C.H.R.).

Brouwer, W. H., Waterink, W., van Wolffelaar, P. C., & Rothengatter, T. (1991). Divided attention in experienced young and older drivers: Lane tracking and visual analysis in a dynamic driving simulator. *Human Factors, 33,* 573–582.

Brown, J., Greaney, K., Mitchel, J., & Lee, W. S. (1993). *Predicting accidents and insurance claims among older drivers.* Southington, CT: ITT Hartford Insurance Group.

Bullough, J. D., Fu, Z., & van Derlofske, J. (2002). *Discomfort and disability glare from halogen and HID headlamp systems* (SAE Technical Paper Series, No. 2002-01-0010). Society of Automotive Engineers.

Chapman, B. G. (1995). Driving with the bioptic. *Journal of Vision Rehabilitation, 9*(4), 19–22.

Cohen, J., & Waiss, B. (1993). An overview of enhancement techniques for peripheral field loss. *Journal of the American Optometric Association, 64,* 60–70.

Colsher, P. L., & Wallace, R. B. (1993). Geriatric assessment and driver functioning. *Clinics in Geriatric Medicine, 9,* 365–376.

DeLibero, V. (1995). *Self-appraisal and driving simulator performance in younger and older drivers.* Unpublished manuscript, Touro College, Dix Hills, New York.

Gianutsos, R. (1988). Computer programs for cognitive rehabilitation: Vol. 6. Driving Advisement System [Computer software]. Bayport, NY: Life Science Associates.

Gianutsos, R. (1991). Visual field deficits after brain injury: Computerized screening. *Journal of Behavioral Optometry, 2,* 143–150.

Gianutsos, R. (1994). Driving advisement with the Elemental Driving Simulator (EDS): When less suffices. *Behavior Research Methods, Instruments, & Computers, 26,* 183–186.

Gianutsos, R. (1996). Vision rehabilitation after brain injury. In M. Gentile & S. Schiff (Eds.), *A therapist's guide to the evaluation and treatment of vision dysfunction and low vision* (pp. 321–342). Bethesda, MD: American Occupational Therapy Association.

Gianutsos, R., & Beattie, A. (1992). Elemental driving simulator. In *Proceedings of the Johns Hopkins National Search for Computing Applications to Assist Persons with Disabilities* (pp. 117–120). Los Alamitos, CA: IEEE Computer Society Press.

Gianutsos, R., Campbell, A., Beattie, A., & Mandriota, F. J. (1992). A computer-augmented quasi-simulation of the cognitive prerequisites for resumption of driving after brain injury. *Assistive Technology, 4,* 70–86.

Gianutsos, R., & Suchoff, I. B. (1996). Visual fields after brain injury: Management issues for the occupational therapist. In M. Scheiman (Ed.), *Vision: Screening and intervention techniques for occupational therapists* (pp. 333–358). Thorofare, NJ: Slack.

Gottlieb, D. D. (1993). *Enhancing awareness, increasing safety, and returning to driving for patient with visual field loss and neglect.* Neuro-Optometric Rehabilitation Association, International annual meeting.

Gottlieb, D. D., Freeman, P., & Williams, M. (1992). Clinical research and statistical analysis of a visual field awareness system. *Journal of the American Optometric Association, 63,* 581–588.

Hall, C. (1995). *Functional visual fields: Norms for younger and older viewers.* Unpublished manuscript, Touro College, Dix Hills, New York.

Johnson, C. A., & Keltner, J. L. (1983). Incidence of visual field loss in 20,000 eyes and its relationship to driving performance. *Archives of Ophthalmology, 101,* 371–375.

Mitchell, S. (1994, October 20). *Brain injury and memory deficits in driver rehabilitation.* In Albany, NY: Northeast Association of Driver Educator's for the Disabled.

Nouri, F. M., Tinson, D. J., & Lincoln, N. B. (1987). Cognitive ability and driving after stroke. *International Disability Studies, 9,* 110–115.

Owsley, C., & Ball, K. (1993). Assessing visual function in the older driver. *Clinics in Geriatric Medicine, 9,* 389–401.

Owsley, C., Ball, K., Sloane, M. E., Roenker, D. L., & Bruni, J. R. (1991). Visual/cognitive correlates of vehicle accidents in older drivers. *Psychology and Aging, 6,* 403–415.

Parasuraman, R., & Nestor, P. (1993). Attention and driving: Assessment in elderly individuals with dementia. *Clinics in Geriatric Medicine, 9,* 377–388.

Parisi, J. L., Bell, R. A., & Yassein, H. (1991). Homonymous hemianopic field defects and driving in Canada. *Canadian Journal of Ophthalmology, 26,* 252–256.

Ramsey, W. E. (1990). Low vision and driving. In *Driving instruction course: Focus on the handicapped.* Presentation given in College Park, MD, and sponsored by the American Automobile Association.

Schiff, W., Arnone, W., & Cross, S. (1994). Driving assessment with computer-video scenarios: More is sometimes better. *Behavior Research Methods, Instruments, and Computers, 26,* 192–194.

Shinar, D., & Scheiber, F. (1991). Visual requirements for safety and mobility of older drivers. *Human Factors, 33,* 507–519.

Strano, C. M. (1989). Effects of visual deficits on ability to drive in traumatically brain-injured population. *Journal of Head Trauma Rehabilitation, 4*(2), 35–43.

Subcommittee on Driver Evaluation and Training for Individuals with Disabilities. (1993). *Final report*. Albany: New York State Vocational and Educational Services for Individuals with Disabilities.

Suter, P. S. (1995). Rehabilitation and management of visual dysfunction following traumatic brain injury. In M. J. Ashley & D. K. Krych (Eds.), *Traumatic brain injury rehabilitation* (pp. 198–220). Boca Raton, FL: CRC Press.

Szlyk, J. P., Brigell, M., & Seiple, W. (1993). Effects of age and hemianopic visual field loss on driving. *Optometry and Vision Science, 70,* 1031–1037.

van Zomeren, A. H., Brouwer, W. H., & Minderhoud, J. M. (1987). Acquired brain damage and driving: A review. *Archives of Physical Medicine and Rehabilitation, 68,* 697–705.

Wang, C. C., Kosinski, C. J., Schwartzbert, J. G., & Shanklin, A. V. (2003). *Physician's guide to assessing and counseling older drivers.* Washington, DC: National Highway Traffic Safety Administration. July 26, 2005, from http://www.ama-assn.org/ama/pub/category/10791.html

West, C. G., et al. (2003). Vision and driving self-restriction in older adults. *Journal of the American Geriatric Society, 51,* 1499–1501.

Wood, J. M. (1993). Can driving performance be predicted by vision testing? [Abstract]. *Optometry and Vision Science, 70,* 134.

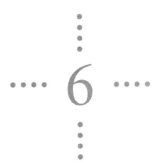

Occupational Therapy and Collaborative Interventions for Adults With Low Vision

Tressa Kern, MS, OTR
Nancy D. Miller, MSW

A challenge for occupational therapists is to use their existing talents and training in working with people with low vision—whether vision impairment is the primary or secondary disability—while a comprehensive knowledge base, integrating scientific, medical, practical, and research wisdom is developed specifically for occupational therapists. Three seminal works (Gentile, 1997; Warren, 2000; American Occupational Therapy Association [AOTA], 2001) have broadened the knowledge base. These works, however, are just the beginning of this ongoing process. In this chapter, the term *low vision* is used to refer to the full continuum of vision loss, from partial sight, to legal blindness, to light perception only.

According to the American Foundation for the Blind (AFB), there are approximately 10 million blind and visually impaired people in the United States, and approximately 1.3 million Americans are legally blind (AFB, 2000). According to AFB, the prevalence of severe vision impairment is age related, and 1 in 6 Americans ages 65 and older experience severe vision loss. Approximately 5.5 million elderly individuals ages 65 and older are blind or visually impaired. By age 85, 1 in 3 older people experience problems with vision that drastically affect the ability to do everyday tasks (AFB, 1999).

A recent report by the National Center for Policy Research for Women and Families, titled "Blind Adults in America: Their Lives and Challenges" (Zuckerman, 2004), stated that most blind adults are older than the general population. Their average age is 62, and 1 out of every 3 is older than age 75. More than three-quarters (more than 79%) are White, 12% are Black, and 6% are Hispanic. The average number of years of education is

11.4. Most blind adults live in an urban area (78%). More (35%) live in the South than in any other geographic area. One in 5 blind men lives alone but that number decreases after age 74. In contrast, blind women are more likely to live alone as they get older, and the majority live alone after age 75. Nearly 1 in 5 blind adults (19%) lives in poverty, a higher percentage than in the general population. Only 19% are currently employed. Very few blind adults report receiving therapy of any kind. Almost half of blind adults receive Social Security or disability benefits, but even they are more likely to live below the poverty line than other adults are. Very few blind adults, including those who are eligible, receive public assistance or food stamps. Most blind adults were not born blind but instead became blind as a result of adult-onset diseases, not accidents. Research shows that prevention and treatment of diabetes, cataracts, and glaucoma could reduce blindness in a substantial number of Americans. Copies of this report are available for free online at http://www.center4policy.org.

Practically all individuals with low vision, even people with legal blindness, can benefit from a low vision examination, prescription of devices, environmental modifications, vision rehabilitation services, or some combination of these.

It is of greatest importance that occupational therapists familiarize themselves with the existing research and literature in low vision, blindness, and vision rehabilitation. Resources for obtaining up-to-date information include journals (i.e., the *Journal of Visual Impairment and Blindness, Journal of Vision Rehabilitation,* the Association for the Education and Rehabilitation of the Blind and Visually Impaired's *Re-View*) and other literature in the fields of vision rehabilitation, adult services, and aging. Some examples are Duffy (2002), Orr (1992) Orr and Rogers (2002), Ringgold (1991), and publications from AWARE Associates for World Action in Rehabilitation and Education (see Appendix 6.A).

The protocols and knowledge base presented in this chapter were developed to provide vision rehabilitation in home and community settings, but they can easily be applied in any setting (e.g., hospital, rehabilitation center, nursing home, adult day care center).

In the United States, the definition of *legal blindness* is central visual acuity of 20/200 or less in the better eye with optimal corrective glasses or a visual field of 20° or less in diameter. This means that a person who is legally blind can identify at 20 ft (~6 m) what a person with normal vision can see at 200 ft (~60 m) away or that the field of vision is limited or restricted to a small area. Being blind does not necessarily mean having no vision. People who are classified as *functionally blind* may have a visual acuity better than 20/200 corrected in the better eye, but because of various conditions (e.g., lack of contrast sensitivity) cannot read ordinary print or function without adaptations. This group of people frequently uses low vision aids such as magnifiers, closed-circuit television, and task lighting. *Vision impairment* is defined as having 20/40 or worse vision in the better eye even with prescription eyeglasses. Regardless of degree of vision loss, using any remaining (residual) vision rarely does further damage.

The term *legal blindness* has been used since 1935 to determine eligibility for a variety of governmental and private benefits and services for people with low vision. Recent publications, practice experience, and research emphasize that functional vision assessments rather than isolated clinical measurements of distance vision, provide more relevant information about an individual's ability to use his or her vision in daily life. Currently, the term *low vision* is used to describe individuals who are neither totally blind nor fully sighted and who may or may not meet the clinical criteria for legal blindness but whose residual vision cannot be corrected to normal with regular eyeglasses or contact lenses. What represents usable vision depends not only on visual functions that are clinically measured but also on the person's ability, motivation, and life circumstances. Low vision can be considered any condition in which a person's visual function is not adequate for his or her visual needs.

People with *congenital blindness,* that is, blindness from birth or shortly thereafter, have no previous visual experience. There are a wide range of learning styles and a variety of differences in personal and experiential backgrounds and, therefore, in levels of concept and language development. For example, congenitally blind people may use, or appear to comprehend, words and concepts that they may not actually understand because of limited real life experiences (e.g., colors).

People with *adventitious blindness* have lost their sight after visual maturation. Having sight memory, adventitiously blind individuals will often draw from their background and life experiences in adapting to vision loss.

Implications of Low Vision

The roots of low vision care for people with partial sight were established at the beginning of the 20th century. The first devices were developed in 1908, when magnifiers were created. Optometrists and ophthalmologists began prescribing magnifiers and telescopes in the 1920s. The first optometric clinic for low vision was opened in 1953 at the Industrial Home for the Blind (now known as Helen Keller Services) in Brooklyn, New York. In the same year, the first ophthalmologic clinic for low vision was founded at the New York Association for the Blind in New York City (now known as *Lighthouse International*). In the 1960s, the first use of advanced technology to provide magnification for people with low vision came with the development of closed-circuit television, which projected magnified text onto a screen.

To best serve a person with low vision, the occupational therapist should incorporate medical research on the effects of various diseases on visual ability while assessing and then ameliorating the disability through rehabilitation. In the ideal situation, after an eye disease has been diagnosed and addressed medically, the next step should be a low vision evaluation by a qualified low vision optometrist or ophthalmologist. It should be recognized that this evaluation is not part of the traditional medical system familiar to occupational therapists.

To find a low vision specialist in your area, you can contact the American Optometric Association, located in St. Louis, Missouri, at 1-800-365-2219, or you can contact the American Academy of Ophthalmology, located in San Francisco, California, at 415-561-8500.

A thorough low vision examination will include, but is not limited to, the following:

- A detailed medical and vision history plus the history of the present impairment or pathology;
- A social history including education level, employment history, hobbies, interest inventory, interpersonal relationships, and socialization choices;
- Self-reported difficulties with activities of daily living (ADL), mobility, and environmental challenges;
- Distance visual acuity, including preferred gaze position and best lighting environment (conditions and contrast for optimal vision function);
- A standard evaluation of accommodation (focusing), pupils, muscle efficiency, balance, color, and stereo vision;
- Keratometry (measure of the curvature of the exterior cornea) and retinoscopy (examination of the retina);
- Manifest refraction (determining the appropriate lens power) and telescopic refraction (use of telescopic devices, if appropriate);
- A comprehensive eye health evaluation, such as tonometry, biomicroscopy, dilated fundus evaluation, and assessment of visual fields;
- An evaluation of near vision; and
- A review of desired goals to be achieved with corrected vision.

The summary of the low vision evaluation may include an optical prescription for distance and near viewing. It also may include a prescription for tints, filters, telescopes, prisms, special lighting, stand or hand magnifiers, and other optical and nonoptical devices. Finally, recommendations for follow-up and monitoring for changes in visual status will be included, when appropriate.

Standardized tools for assessing vision function are used by optometrists and ophthalmologists, including those with specialized training in low vision, as part of the low vision examination. Examples of the most commonly used assessment tools (e.g., Hirschberg Test, Polaroid Tests, Worth 4 Dot Test) can be found in Anderson (1982), Duane (1990), and Faye (1984). The best way to learn how to read a low vision examination report is to consult with a low vision optometrist or ophthalmologist and actually review a clinical low vision examination report together. This exercise not only will enable the occupational therapist to become familiar with the vocabulary but also will also result in a better understanding of the clinical measures and their value. In addition, it is extremely informative to observe a clinical low vision examination.

Vision Rehabilitation System for Serving People Who Are Blind or Visually Impaired

The low vision and blindness system comprises a network of services provided by government, educational, and not-for-profit agencies serving people with low vision. Major funding is appropriated through the federal Rehabilitation Act of 1973, Public Law 93-112, 29 USC 701 et seq, and its amendments Public Law 95-602, HR 12467, H Rept 95-1149, as well as other federal, state, or local programs and private dollars, including foundations. Numerous private voluntary agencies, state agencies, and consumer groups also deliver services for people with low vision or total blindness. Services differ greatly from one state or community to another. Each state organizes the service delivery system for vision rehabilitation differently. The structure of service delivery is influenced by the state's history of services, resources, and philosophy. Some states, such as New York, have designated state agencies or departments serving people who are legally blind, with another agency serving people with vision impairments. One of the best ways to identify and access services for a person with vision loss in a particular state is to consult the AFB *Directory of Services,* available online at http://www.afb.org (or call toll-free, 1-800-AFB-LINE [1-800-232-5463] for a list of local service providers).

Veterans who are blind and visually impaired receive comprehensive services from the Department of Veterans Affairs. The health care system is a third resource for funding vision rehabilitation.

According to the American Occupational Therapy Association's *Practice Guidelines for Adults With Low Vision* (Warren, 2001), delivery of low vision rehabilitation services through the health care system is not as well established as that of the blindness system.

Since 1990, coverage by Medicare Part B for occupational therapy services for individuals with primary vision loss can be accessed. This is a result of the Health Care Financing Administration's (now called the Centers for Medicare and Medicaid Services) expansion of the definition of *physical disabilities* to include vision impairment. Occupational therapy services can be provided when prescribed by a physician. This expanded definition is due in large part to the efforts of ophthalmologists such as Donald Fletcher. As a result, hospitals, clinics, and rehabilitation facilities are moving toward including low vision and vision rehabilitation programs as part of their services.

The Balanced Budget Refinement Act of 1999, Public Law 106-113, further validated the role of occupational therapists in treating Medicare patients with low vision by authorizing optometrists to refer patients to occupational therapists beginning January 1, 2000 (Warren, 2001).

In 2002, the Centers for Medicare and Medicaid Services (CMS) published a program memorandum alerting physicians and the provider community that Medicare beneficiaries who are blind and visually impaired are eligible for physician-prescribed rehabilitation services from approved health care professionals on the same basis as beneficiaries with other medical conditions that result in reduced physical functioning (CMS, 2002).

Recently, vision rehabilitation professionals (e.g., rehabilitation teachers [RTs] and orientation and mobility [O&M] specialists) have been billing Medicare for services with a written treatment plan established by a medical physician (which may be an optometrist or ophthalmologist) and implemented by an approved Medicare provider. However, each local Medicare carrier determines whether this is allowed and under which ICD codes the service may be billed.

In 2004, Congress legislated a 1-year study to produce recommendations for legislative or administrative action providing for the payment for vision rehabilitation services by vision rehabilitation professionals, including RTs, O&M specialists, and occupational therapists. The appropriations bill established a 5-year demonstration project, commencing July 1, 2004, to provide standardized national coverage for vision rehabilitation services by vision rehabilitation professionals. This was due in large part to the efforts of the National Vision Rehabilitation Cooperative (now the National Vision Rehabilitation Association).

Other potential funding streams for home-based occupational therapy for people with low vision include foundation grants, as well as county, city, or state grants, secured by not-for-profit agencies for occupational therapy services for people with low vision.

Low Vision Rehabilitation: An Expanding Service Area

Because of the expanding reimbursement options, a person with vision impairment is a desirable patient. Occupational therapists in clinical, home, and community-based settings will see an increasing number of people with vision problems, related to the demographics of an aging society. Dramatic increases are predicted in the over-75 age group in which severe vision loss will affect a large part of the population.

Older people report struggling with the everyday instrumental tasks that are necessary to maintain a household in the community when they experience vision loss. Clear evidence of unmet needs exists (Branch, Horowitz, & Carr, 1989).

The occupational therapist's comprehensive knowledge of the physical, cognitive, sensory, and psychosocial aspects of disability enables him or her to implement interventions that will enhance the outcomes for an individual involved in the process of vision rehabilitation. This is the case when the vision loss is the only disability as well as when it is one of multiple impairments. Most occupational therapists encounter people with multiple impairments for whom vision loss is also present.

It is essential that occupational therapists working with people with low vision and blindness acquire additional specialized knowledge in addition to seeking the partnership of vision rehabilitation professionals. This specialized education should include an understanding of ocular pathology causing vision loss, common treatment procedures, the application of modalities typical in vision rehabilitation, and the spectrum and use of commonly prescribed optical devices. Occupational therapists who are fortunate enough to work directly with optometrists and ophthalmologists specializing in low vision will have the benefit of experiential learning. Occupational therapists should avail themselves of the many resources currently available, including vision rehabilitation journals, textbooks, and online resources, as well as participate in continuing education courses and certificate programs.

Occupational therapists must also become familiar with their counterparts working in the vision rehabilitation system. These professionals primarily include RTs, O&M specialists, and rehabilitation counselors.

History and Role of Rehabilitation Professionals

Three types of professionals with specific expertise comprise the established rehabilitation team providing services for adults and senior citizens with impaired vision: (a) RTs, (b) O&M specialists, and (c) certified rehabilitation counselors (CRCs). Those in each parallel field have an extensive history of professional preparation, expertise, and certification spanning decades, comparable to occupational therapy. Figure 6.1 depicts our view of the role delineation and functions of occupational therapists, RTs, and O&M specialists. In addition, there are, professionals who combine the skills and certifications of RTs and O&M specialists, and also low vision assistants (LVAs), teachers of the visually impaired (TVIs), and low vision therapists (LVTs).

Rehabilitation Teachers

RTs differ from other medical rehabilitation practitioners in that their exclusive emphasis is on the effect of visual impairment on ADLs, on the family, and on the person's life situation. University courses in RT started in the United States in the 1930s, and a full degree program was established in 1963. RT programs throughout the United States confer a master's degree in RT or a master's degree in special education or rehabilitation counseling with an emphasis (concentration or certificate) in RT. Curriculum, practicum, and internship requirements for professional preparation programs are monitored and accredited by the Academy for Certification of Vision Rehabilitation and Education Professionals (ACVREP) in Tucson, Arizona.

RTs work with children (typically not with infants), youth, adults, and senior citizens. They teach many specialized adaptive and alternative skills, such as the following:
- *Communication:* use of Braille, sensory development and listening skills, adaptations for reading and writing, abacus, mathematical systems, and computer use;
- *Personal management:* clothing care and grooming, medication management, child care, eating, and social skills;
- *Home management:* meal preparation, home mechanics, marking and labeling systems, record keeping, and safety procedures;
- *Leisure activities:* hobbies, games, hand crafts, and accessing community activities;

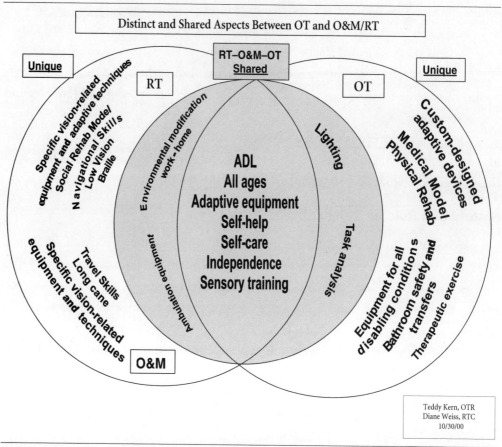

Figure 6.1. RT–O&M–OT areas of practice shared.
Note. RT = rehabilitation teacher; O&M = orientation and mobility specialist; OT = occupational therapist; ADL = activities of daily living.

- *Orientation and movement* within the home or facility;
- *Training in the use of optical devices:* magnifiers, telescopes, closed-circuit television, image enhancers, and similar prescribed devices;
- *Training in the use of assistive devices* specific to low vision or total blindness;
- *Guidance and counseling:* adaptation to vision loss and encouraging family support.

Some skill areas overlap between occupational therapists and RTs. Both professions teach people to appropriately use all of their remaining physical capacity and senses and how to analyze and organize tasks and situations for maximum independence in daily living. RTs' comprehensive approach uses specialized training and knowledge of alternative methods, technology, and devices used by children, youth, adults, and senior citizens with vision loss.

Orientation and Mobility Specialists

O&M specialists teach individuals how to orient themselves to the layout of their home; immediate environment; neighborhood; workplace; and the community in general, including street crossings and use of public transportation. Training also is provided in basic sighted-guide and self-protection techniques or long-cane skills for independent travel needs.

For people with low vision and blindness, a challenge is to gather auditory, tactile, and other sensory data that will keep them oriented. The next task is to learn to protect themselves by mastering techniques to guard against hazards such as stairs; curbs; vehicles; and edges of subway, bus, or train platforms. O&M specialists teach these skills to people of all ages from infants (pre-cane) to senior citizens.

In the 1950s, the numbers of veterans with vision impairments returning from World War II prompted the development of long-cane travel and mobility techniques. Master's-level university programs to train O&M professionals began in 1961. Personnel preparation and continuing education are offered through universities and AER. Professional certification is offered through the ACVREP.

Orientation techniques enable travelers to use sensory information to establish their position in space. Individuals learn to identify their location in the physical environment, determine their proximity to significant objects, and gain awareness of surface changes. Mobility techniques for people with low vision and blindness are designed to teach them how to travel safely and independently from one location to another, indoors and outdoors. They may learn to use one or more of the following: long canes, the sighted-guide technique, electronic travel aids, dog guides, and prescribed optical devices. O&M specialists also teach the interpretation of sounds and other environmental cues (e.g., odors, vibrations, wind, temperature) for people with vision loss to help create a mental map while the individual learns how to remain alert to danger signals.

Dually Trained Professionals

A new type of professional is emerging that combines the skills and certifications of RTs and O&M specialists. These professionals have dual certification and training in both O&M and RT and take two examinations from the ACVREP for certification. Dually trained professionals currently practice primarily in New York State but are expanding their practice nationwide. Several universities offer dual training programs including Hunter College of the City University of New York in New York.

Certified Rehabilitation Counselors

CRCs not only provide counseling specific to occupation and employment goals but also administer vocational interest inventories, offer career guidance, and teach interviewing and on-the-job skills. CRCs introduce workplace technology; facilitate job placement; develop referral relationships with employers; and assist with planning, interviewing, and adjusting to work and the workplace. In some rehabilitation agencies, the CRC is the intake coordinator and case manager, whereas in other agencies, a social worker performs that function. CRCs are increasingly involved in transition planning for youth with blindness and low vision from school to work and in prevocational services for preteens and young adults.

In some states, CRCs can take a state examination to become state certified, and professional certification is available from the Commission on Rehabilitation Counselors Certification in Rolling Meadows, Illinois.

Low Vision Assistants, Teachers of the Visually Impaired, and Low Vision Therapists

In addition to the primary professionals listed above, people with blindness and low vision also receive service from, or may encounter, *LVAs, TVIs,* and *LVTs.* LVAs and LVTs, who are certified specialists, describe and demonstrate optical and nonoptical aids, teach people the proper use and maintenance of prescribed devices, and generally work in a clinical setting with ophthalmologists or optometrists. They teach eccentric viewing techniques and the use of peripheral vision. This instruction has become an integral part of low vision care.

TVIs are certified in elementary or secondary education. They are not tutors in special subject areas (i.e., math, foreign languages), but rather they address the expanded core curricular areas unique to vision impairment. TVIs work with ages from infancy to high school graduation. They specialize, with academic subject teachers, in ways to adapt the presentation of information and the use of alternative strategies and materials in public, private, and residential school settings.

Occupational Therapists' Role in the Multidisciplinary Team

It is important for occupational therapists to intervene and participate in the rehabilitation process for individuals with blindness and low vision in the following cases:
- When an additional functional limitation exists or a physical condition affects the individual with low vision;
- When a person with low vision or blindness ages with concomitant sensory, physical, and age-related functional impairments, or both; and
- When a person with multiple impairments ages and exhibits a functional vision impairment.

In the past, occupational therapists would have been unlikely to work with adults or senior citizens with low vision. This was especially true when no further functional impairment or medical condition existed in addition to the vision loss. An occupational therapist was often assigned to work with a person with low vision when an RT was unavailable.

Setting specific occupational therapy goals (VISIONS/Services for the Blind and Visually Impaired, 2000) for people with low vision or blindness must include a discussion of the individual's level of function before diagnosis and, subsequently, a treatment plan to improve the person's current functional skills and quality of life by doing the following:

- Determining the person's previous functional ADL level and other productive activities before vision loss;
- Determining family relations, work history, and level of social interaction affecting function;
- Evaluating performance capacities and deficits in visual and physical function in the person's own home and community environment, for example, evaluating safety in bathing activities, eating and dressing skills, communications, and personal and financial management;
- Establishing a comprehensive treatment plan that takes into account the physical, cognitive, sensorineural, and vision limitations affecting the person;
- Establishing, along with the person, his or her specific goals, which may include functional skills in ADL, indoor travel, and restoration of physical function in which a deficit or impairment is determined, and then applying behavioral objectives in developing treatment plans;
- Selecting tasks, activities, or exercises appropriate to achieve defined needs and objectives and facilitating learning through a variety of vision rehabilitation techniques to achieve desired outcomes;
- Teaching specific sensorimotor activities, exercises, and postural alignment techniques to improve gait and navigational skills in preparation for O&M training;
- Devising, designing, or selecting assistive devices specific to vision loss or equipment related to ADL needs;
- Evaluating response and progress;
- Assessing and measuring change and development of functional independence;
- Sharing findings and their relevance to other professionals and assistants in the vision rehabilitation team; and
- Collaborating with RTs and O&M professionals to enable the person with blindness or low vision to achieve his or her maximum level of independent functioning.

Goal-oriented teaching techniques are used to meet the behavioral objectives and will vary depending on the person's level of physical and cognitive ability and sensory function in addition to vision loss.

The occupational therapist traditionally provides training in ADLs (e.g., eating, dressing, grooming, toileting), transfers and positioning, splinting, energy conservation, work simplification techniques, environmental modifications, increasing range of motion, strength training, endurance for completion of tasks, and fine motor coordination. The RT may be qualified to teach some, but certainly not all, of these techniques.

The importance of the occupational therapist intervening and participating in the rehabilitation process for individuals with low vision is based on the unique expertise that occupational therapists provide in teaching adaptive living skills, the use of adaptive equipment, and in modifying the physical environment. Current rehabilitation practices and blindness-based rehabilitation services for people with low vision sometimes overlook or fail to recognize the valuable expertise the occupational therapist brings to the rehabilitation process (Kern, 1996). Occupational therapists themselves may circumvent or avoid working with people with blindness or low vision because of limited experience, education, or exposure to people with this disability. Occupational therapists must take advantage of the increasing opportunities for continuing education. For example, there are workshops and seminars sponsored by AOTA and continuing education seminars by AER (see Appendix 6.A).

In any interdisciplinary relationship, each colleague brings to the experience a particular expertise. Specifically in the rehabilitation of people with blindness and low vision, an occupational therapist brings a medically based body of knowledge but lacks the specific hands-on knowledge of blindness or low vision. Similarly, the RT, O&M specialist, and LVT, whose backgrounds are specific to blindness, have a vision-related medical education and a limited ability to comprehensively assess performance capacities and functional disabilities unrelated to blindness.

A growing number of occupational therapists working primarily in vision rehabilitation settings have completed specific training that qualifies them to assume the function of an RT. For example, Lighthouse International in New York City offers an RT training program that qualifies the graduate to take the ACVREP certification examination. This training has attracted occupational therapists as well as other professionals seeking specialized training.

It is important to acknowledge the common philosophical base between these disciplines. In occupational therapy, there is a general assumption that "the goal is to achieve a person–environment fit that enables the older person to function as competently as possible" (Rogers, 1981, p. 664). Like occupational therapy, the vision rehabilitation system operates on the assumption that independence goals are determined with the person served and not solely by the professional. All of the disciplines use life experience as part of the therapeutic process. The shared knowledge base common to all members of the rehabilitation team is drawn from the principles of andragogy.

Andragogy is the study and implementation of conditions relevant to adult learning. The learning is problem centered and is a process for problem finding and solving in the present. Andragological principles lead to the creation of a self-directed adult learning environment in which there is reciprocity in the teaching–learning relationship—a helping, rather than a directing, relationship. "According to the principles of androgogy, the student is an autonomous adult, functioning within his/her own highly developed world of values, interests and attitudes" (Phillips & Correia, 1979, p. 11).

Whenever a multidisciplinary, interdisciplinary, or transdisciplinary approach is used, many concerns must be addressed, including

- Overcoming differences in vocabulary usage by various disciplines,
- Developing methods for managing conflicting recommendations,
- Supporting role sharing and role release (a transdisciplinary approach),
- Minimizing territoriality and competition for the same population,
- Acknowledging differences in reimbursement or competition for the same dollars, and
- Ensuring methods for developing shared goals between professionals and with the visually impaired person.

The collaboration between occupational therapists and other professionals in the field of vision rehabilitation services can take place in work settings where occupational therapists are on staff with RTs, O&M specialists, CRCs, and LVIs. Occupational therapists may be included on a consultant basis by a vision rehabilitation agency or by a state commission for people with blindness or low vision.

One reason for the greater involvement with people with visual impairments is that many of the specialists who customarily provide vision rehabilitation are not available in less populated or rural areas, where the universally prevalent rehabilitation specialists are physical therapists and occupational therapists.

An essential resource to understanding the evolving role of occupational therapists in working with people with low vision is AOTA's (2001) *Occupational Therapy Practice Guidelines for Adults With Low Vision*.

Tools for Occupational Therapists Who Work With People With Low Vision

Vision Screening Checklist

Traditionally educated occupational therapists are not professionally trained to conduct low vision evaluations or to recommend the use and application of prescribed low vision aids (e.g., telescopes, binocular magnifiers). However, it is important that occupational therapists learn about these functions and how to integrate a functional vision assessment into their existing evaluation process. The ideal time to administer such a checklist is prior to the first treatment session, following medical intake. A private setting is recommended to gather the most candid responses. One tool that has proven to be useful in facilitating an informal assessment of functional vision, applicable in any setting (e.g., home, clinic, day care) is a functional vision screening checklist, such as the example that follows.

Be aware that it is important to the adequate completion of any self-reported survey to incorporate direct questions and to elicit anecdotal information that goes beyond the clinical diagnosis. Simple, straightforward questions elicit the best responses. A format and some examples of questions that can be included on a functional vision screening checklist include those in Exhibit 6.1.

Exhibit 6.1. Sample Questions on a Functional Vision Screening Checklist

To prepare a functional vision screening checklist, gather in advance an 8.5 × 11 in. (21.6 cm × 28 cm) sheet of heavyweight white, unlined paper with 1-in. (2.5 cm) size numbers, evenly spaced (not close together), written with a black, bold marker. Four numbers are adequate on the page. On a second sheet, write smaller numbers (0.5 in. [1.3 cm]) evenly spaced, six on a page.

- Do you have trouble seeing?
- How long have you experienced this difficulty?
- Do you know the cause? Has an eye doctor diagnosed or treated you?
- Which eye is affected most?
- What *can* you see? Is it blurry or clear?
  - Headlines of a newspaper?
  - Newsprint?
  - Details on a television screen?
  - Food on your plate?
  - Stoplights and street signs?
- Do you see better straight ahead (central vision) or if you look to one side (peripheral vision)?
- Can you see the color red (bright color)? What color am I wearing?
- Does lighting make a difference? Does bright light help?
- Does glare (e.g., from the sun, reflected light) bother you? Indoor glare? Outdoor glare?
- What activities were you doing for yourself before your vision problem interfered (e.g., housecleaning, cooking, shopping, laundry, reading, and independent travel)? What about now?
- Can you read these numbers? (Display the "number" pages you created, first the 1 in. [2.5 cm], then the 0.5 in. [1.3 cm]; allow the person to hold the page as close as necessary to be able to see it.)
- When you are walking outdoors, do you depend on others, or do you rely on your own vision? How do you know when to cross the street?
- Does your vision change from day to day, or during different times of the day?
- Describe any special glasses or devices you use to see better (e.g., optical aids). Where did you get them?
- When did you have your last eye exam?
- What is your eye doctor's name?

Occupational therapy practitioners must begin to develop their own tools for assessing vision function as it applies to the medical model. Until standard occupational therapy tools are formalized, it would be prudent to integrate a functional vision screening checklist. According to Mary Warren (1995),

> If occupational therapy is to make a unique and lasting contribution to this practice area, we must develop our own frame of reference for addressing the needs of persons with low vision that must be compatible with our other theories regarding adaptation to disease and environment, and must go beyond merely advocating the use of adaptive devices and techniques. Our frame of reference must focus, in part, on how the central nervous system is best able to adapt to a loss in one of its major information gathering systems. (pp. 858–859)

Screening for Physical and Occupational Therapy Referral

One of the most useful screening, assessment, and curriculum instruments for identifying the need for occupational therapy was developed by therapists at the Alabama Institute for Deaf and Blind, to be used by any service professional. The Screening for Physical and Occupational Therapy Referral (SPOTR), developed through a National Independent Living Skills grant project, was designed to provide an objective, cost-effective method of referral for evaluation, therapy, or other services for individuals ages 16 years and older with sensory loss. The SPOTR is based on a fundamental belief in a multidisciplinary approach to evaluation and training of independent-living skills. Because it is designed specifically to be used with a population that is visually impaired, hearing impaired, or both, it is a particularly useful and unique assessment tool. Until recently, most assessment tools have been inappropriate for this population because of the lack of normative data, strict standardization, and tests, which depend on visual skills (Woosley, Harden, & Murphy, 1983).

Collaboration

Until such time as the complete scientific base is established and communicated to all occupational therapists, the current standard of practice for people with low vision should include collaboration with vision rehabilitation disciplines and practitioners. These include ophthalmologists, optometrists, RTs, O&M specialists, LVTs, and CRCs.

Low vision rehabilitation as a distinct practice area within occupational therapy still lacks the specific experience, training, and techniques used by O&M specialists and RTs. Even without specialized training, however, an occupational therapist can use familiar problem-solving skills to assist a person with low vision. For example, basic ADL skills training using greater or lesser adaptations for visual functioning is still needed. It must be understood that training will take longer as the person with low vision learns compensatory techniques that are specific to his or her remaining visual function.

Evaluation

A comprehensive low vision evaluation requires specific, specialized knowledge of vision and low vision, with education and training in optometry, ophthalmology, and the low vision rehabilitation field. Clinical measures of visual skills, however, provide only fundamental information about a person's vision. The measures are incomplete and do not represent a complete picture of the individual. The functional effect of a visual impairment is likely to be best measured outside the clinic, preferably in the home environment. Some system for doing so needs to be built into every service program (Orr, 1992).

Occupational therapists must consider the functional implications of the eye condition as well as the person's motivation and the degree to which he or she understands and accepts the impairment. Also important to take into account is the degree to which the vision impairment interferes with the person's goals for functional independence (Lampert & Lapolice, 1995). Once the person's desires and capabilities are taken into account, the occupational therapist must apply this knowledge to the evaluation process.

Adaptations for visual functioning include attention to color contrast; lighting (including reduced glare); placement of objects; use of cognitive, muscle, and motor memory in lieu of vision; and use of residual vision. A functional assessment through interview and observation can and should always include the observation of visual skills in the performance of self-care and homemaking tasks. For example, reading ability, which in many situations might be thought of as leisure activity, influences a person's ability to maintain independence, that is, through reading labels, written instructions, appliance dials and controls, timepieces and watches, thermostats, mail and correspondence, telephone numbers, and telephone dials.

Task Analysis

In addition to using a vision screening tool and completing a traditional evaluation, the therapist needs to focus on the functional impact of the vision loss on ADL. One way of accomplishing this is through *task analysis*.

An example of a functional task analysis familiar to occupational therapists, which may be useful in both clinical and home-based environments, is the task of telephone dialing as a measure of both physical and visual status (AFB, 1972). This task incorporates the use of central vision, sensory integration skills, manual dexterity, eye–hand coordination, and proprioceptive and kinesthetic abilities. The examiner should use a standard telephone or telephone dial overlay (available for both rotary and touch-tone phones that are not hand held) for use in the assessment. Overlays are available free of charge from the local telephone company for people with special needs. In addition, a large-numeral telephone should be available nearby. See Exhibits 6.2 and 6.3 for techniques and integrating skills in task analysis.

Exhibit 6.2. Techniques in Task Analysis

- Place a rotary or touch-tone telephone on a table in front of the visually impaired person. Ask whether he or she can see it, and ask him or her to dial his or her own telephone number, if possible, or 911, or "0" for the operator.
- Observe how the person reaches for the telephone. Does he or she grope and search, or immediately locate the receiver?
- Ask "Can you see the number?" Ask the person to find the number "5" (middle of the dial). Can he or she dial in a timely manner? If not, can the person trail his or her fingers in a circular movement (on a rotary dial) or line by line (on a touch-tone telephone) to locate numbers?
- If the person has difficulty dialing a number or locating a reference number, ask him or her to locate "0" for the operator. If placement of fingers on the dial or touch-tone pad of the telephone is difficult because of arthritis, neuropathy, or another upper-extremity condition, this should be noted and distinguished from the visual process.

Exhibit 6.3. Integrating Skills in Task Analysis

- Can the person hold the receiver? Can he or she coordinate dialing and holding receiver? Can the person directly return receiver to the cradle? Does he or she use vision, or visual scanning techniques, or is it necessary to use both hands to search to accomplish this task? Do verbal instructions help? Tactual cues? If the person exhibits difficulty, place a large-print telephone dial overlay onto the telephone (or use a big-button, large-numeral telephone) and repeat the evaluation.
- Note the lighting conditions during the administration of the task analysis. Does increasing the illumination (e.g., using a higher wattage bulb) or changing the position of the light source (e.g., moving it directly over the telephone as task lighting) improve the person's performance of the task? In practice, illumination preferences and needs are highly individual. The visually impaired person himself or herself is the best guide for information on helpfulness and comfort with types and levels of lighting.
- Other tasks, such as personal grooming and dressing, can be analyzed in the same way to develop the comprehensive treatment plan.

Treatment Considerations Based on Vision Rehabilitation Techniques

Functional vision loss is defined as "how the vision deficit effects [*sic*] the person's ability to function in the performance of their usual tasks" (Fox & Kern, 1992, p. 5.) Once a functional vision assessment is completed, it is important to include in the treatment plan methods to help the person adapt to vision loss through environmental and behavioral techniques. Maximizing the use of residual vision will include consideration of the following:

- Lighting (e.g., overhead, body level, natural, and artificial);
- Contrast;
- Glare;
- Preferred field of view (e.g., best gaze posture);
- Adaptations of reading materials (e.g., print size, color, fatigue factors, time needed for recognition); and
- Use of large print, braille, or recorded media.

Important for the person are recommendations for nonprescriptive optical aids such as bold-line paper, specialized pens, reading stands, and writing guides. These aids and many others are available through specialized Web sites, catalogs, vendors, and some vision rehabilitation agencies. However, insurance (HMOs or PPOs) rarely covers the cost of nonoptical devices and aids. The commission or department for blindness services in the particular state of residence may cover the cost of devices and aids as well as training in how to use them.

A comprehensive treatment plan must also take into account the following environmental factors (especially in the kitchen, bathroom, and living area in private homes; and the cafeteria, bathrooms, lounge, hallways, and entries in other facilities):

- Object and room dimension (e.g., shape, size, doorways)
- Architectural variations (e.g., corners, floor-to-wall transitions, whether doors are closed or open, whether the floor is carpeted or bare)
- Placement and height of objects (e.g., at body level, overhanging, near or far)
- Signage (e.g., names and numbers on doors, directional indicators)
- Lighting (e.g., optimal illumination without glare, overhead lights, floor lamps, table lamps, task lights, incandescent [preferred], fluorescent, window coverings, wattage of light bulbs, reflection, presence of natural light, lighting of stairwells and landings)
- Furnishings (e.g., texture for tactile clues, patterns that are confusing)
- Use of color contrast (e.g., light objects against dark backgrounds, dark objects against light backgrounds, same-color doors and frames that contrast with walls, doorknobs or handles that contrast with door colors, color edging of steps and ramps)
- Signage (e.g., at eye level, size of print, location).

Instructional Materials and Guidelines

Many of the detailed techniques for training adults and senior citizens with vision impairment in daily living skills are available to occupational therapists on the Internet, in books (in print and on cassette), and through publications. Materials are available from VISIONS/Services for the Blind and Visually Impaired-Center for Independent Living Publications Series, Associates for World Action in Rehabilitation and Education

New Independence Publications, and the book *Making Life More Livable: Simple Adaptations for Living at Home After Vision Loss* (Duffy, 2002). Exhibit 6.4 details 19 guidelines that can assist occupational therapists in the evaluation, treatment, and instructional process.

Exhibit 6.4. Guidelines for the Occupational Therapy Evaluation, Treatment, and Instructional Process

1. Identify yourself as soon as you enter the room.
2. Speak directly to the person, not with your back to him or her or directing your conversation to another part of the room.
3. Your speaking voice need not be louder than normal.
4. Let the person know when you are leaving the room.
5. Tell the person what you are going to do before you administer any test assessment or initiate direct contact.
6. Do not be concerned about using words such as *look* or *see*. These are often the simplest words to use to get your point across. Chances are, the person who is visually impaired will use these words as well.
7. Speak directly to the person, never through a companion or caregiver when the person is present.
8. If you must leave the person alone, make sure that he or she is oriented to his or her surroundings or can maintain physical contact with the environment.
9. Use specific words and directions.
10. Avoid expressions such as "over there," "right here," or "straight ahead." These phrases are vague and should be used sparingly.
11. Offer specific directions, such as "Your comb is on the left side of the dresser toward the back." Say "Let me show you," and guide the person to it, or say "Let me take your hand and show you where it is" and place it on the object (hand-over-hand technique). You might say "to your right" or tap the object and say "it is here" to help the person to determine the direction from which the sound originates.
12. Do not be misinformed. Eyes cannot be weakened or damaged by use of residual vision, except with extreme or excessive use leading to eyestrain (i.e., from computer-based activities).
13. Allow enough time to learn the task. Do not rush through lessons.
14. Take into account that the length of time in accomplishing a specific task will be affected by vision loss.
15. Whenever possible, build a clear mental image (word picture) of the object with which you are working and the steps involved in the project before you attempt to teach a skill.

(continued)

Exhibit 6.4. *Continued*

16. Do not be overprotective. How much assistance to provide will be important to assess throughout treatment. Let the person do as much as possible independently. Persons with low vision may create their own techniques suited to their individual needs. Do not prevent a person from using these techniques unless they are unsafe.

17. For better visibility, use 14-point type (or letters that are 1 in. [2.5 cm] in height). This is useful to remember when ordering labels or rewriting telephone numbers.

18. Use a clock reference point to describe the position of food on a plate or items on a table. This is useful when food is served. For example, "Your meat is at 6 o'clock, vegetables at 9 o'clock, and potatoes at 1 o'clock." This is a vision rehabilitation technique to share with family members and caregivers.

19. Be specific when stating that you are putting food, liquid, or any object in front of the person before doing so; let the person know it is there, and identify its exact location in relation to the person.

Activities and Suggested Procedures

The following are a few basic functional activities that people with low vision generally want to do independently and that should be evaluated and addressed by the therapist. These are by no means the only skills that people with low vision will want to address; neither will every person need to focus on all of them. The tasks and the suggested procedures are sample methods for performing each specific function. Personal preferences, physical or sensory impairments other than vision loss, and the habits of the individual will influence the best techniques for teaching these and other skills.

Self-Care Tasks

Self-care tasks include personal grooming, bathing and toileting, nail and hair care, toothpaste application, medication management, cosmetics application, shaving, cleaning, and maintaining eye or limb prostheses.

A sample procedure for toothpaste application would be as follows:

• The person removes the cap from the tube of toothpaste and places it in a familiar and secure location.

• The person grasps the bristles of the toothbrush, which are facing upward, between the thumb and index finger of one hand, making sure the bristle tops are slightly below the holding fingers. (These fingers will become "guides" in determining where to apply toothpaste.)

- The person curls the remaining fingers of that hand around the toothbrush handle.
- With the toothpaste tube in the other hand, place the tip of the tube between the tips of the fingers (guides), which are holding the toothbrush.
- Squeeze the bottom of the tube gently (this may take practice) until the toothpaste only covers the top of the bristles between the finger guides.
- Remove the tube. Place it in a secure location.

After teeth have been brushed or dentures washed, replace the cap on the tube of toothpaste and return the tube to a specified, consistent location. Note that if the person demonstrates difficulty in easily locating his or her mouth, that proprioceptive skill must be addressed.

Eating Skills and Table Behavior

Eating skills and table behavior include the following: seating self at table, use of utensils, setting the table, buffer techniques, using seasoning and condiments, pouring liquids, serving food, cutting and slicing techniques, carrying containers of food or liquid, table orientation, and locating food.

The procedures for filling and pouring containers of hot and cold liquid are similar. However, hot liquids require more care and training. A sample procedure for pouring liquids would be as follows:

- *Finger or tactual method*: Rest the thumb and middle finger gently on opposite edges (inside and outside) of the cup or glass. Use the index finger to locate and guide the spout or container from which you are pouring over the edge of the cup, pouring slowly in spurts, moving the index finger gradually into the cup or glass, and continue pouring until the liquid reaches the tip of the index finger.
- *Weight method*: As experience is gained in pouring and filling, the desired amount of liquid can often be judged by the weight of the cup or glass.

Two very useful adaptive devices are the "Say When" liquid level indicator, available from Lighthouse International or Maxi-Aids, and the HotShot Single Cup Beverage Maker, also available from Maxi-Aids (see Appendix 6.A for contact information).

Food Labeling, Kitchen Skills, and Meal Preparation

Food labeling, kitchen skills, and meal preparation include the following activities: labeling and storing foods; identifying and using utensils, pots, and pans, and appliances (e.g., toaster, broiler oven, microwave, blender, can opener); setting dials; fitting a plug into an outlet; measuring ingredients; regulating gas and electric burners; using a timer; following recipes and cooking instructions; and cutting, chopping, and slicing.

The desired method and amount of labeling of canned and packaged foods will vary with each individual. Some people prefer to have everything labeled, whereas others want very little labeling and prefer to depend on memory. Sample procedures for labeling foods include the following:

- Using a Dymo-Writer to produce labels on plastic strips. This is useful for permanent identification.
- Using rubber bands placed around cans; for example, one rubber band for peaches, two for green beans, and so on.
- Pasting or taping assorted shapes or small objects, such as paper clips or buttons, onto containers, with each having a specific meaning to the person.
- Using other types of everyday labeling materials, including brightly colored plastic or electrical tape, safety pins, pipe cleaners, hook-and-loop fastener dots, velour pads or furniture protectors, and iron-on patches.
- Using plastic lids that are available for storing open cans of food and come in various sizes. Similar techniques can be used for packaged food. The size, shape, and location of packaged foods usually become guides to the contents.
- Using one of the many special marking and labeling products, such as Hi-Marks, 3-D markers, or Spot 'n' Line pens, available from catalogs specializing in products for people with vision loss.
- Using a black, wide-tip marker or laundry marker write in large bold letters on plain white 3 × 5-in. (7.6 × 12.7 cm) index cards. These labels can be used to differentiate household supplies that may be stored in similarly shaped containers, such as window cleaners, bathroom cleaners, and all-purpose cleaners. Attach each card to the appropriate container with a rubber band.

Home Management and Domestic Tasks

Home management and domestic tasks include the following: shopping and reading prices, making shopping lists, washing dishes, basic cleaning skills (e.g., of sinks, countertops, stoves, windows), loading and operating a dishwasher, doing the laundry (e.g., preparing and separating clothes, operating the washing machine and dryer, hand-washing clothes, ironing, identifying and organizing clothing, hanging and separating clothes), needle threading and sewing, packing a suitcase, making a bed, sweeping and using a vacuum cleaner, and performing minor household repairs.

Keeping dishes clean and sanitary is important and requires special attention when visual scanning for cleanliness is compromised. A sample procedure for washing dishes follows:

- To clean glassware and cups, apply detergent to sponge or pad.
- Insert a sponge or nonabrasive cleaning pad into the bottom of the cup or glass. Do not force a hand into the glass, as pressure can break it. Twist the sponge back and forth to remove dried-on food or debris. Place sponge in the sink. Rinse cup or glass thoroughly and place it upside down in a dish drainer or drying rack, or in a secure location.
- Wash both the front and back of plates and bowls thoroughly; use a wet sponge or cleaning pad to remove dried-on foods, using a repeated circular motion. Place the plate or bowl into the sink and rinse thoroughly, then place into a drainer to dry.

- Keep all sharp knives and pointed kitchen forks or other sharp utensils in one consistent location in the sink, and wash them separately from other utensils. Rinse them with hot water. Always place utensils with sharp ends down in a dish or utensil drainer to dry.

Communications Skills and Money Management

Communications skills and money management include the following activities: using a tape recorder; using a reading machine, computer, or calculator; using a telephone; writing a signature and making out and signing checks or money orders; addressing and mailing bills; keeping financial records; reading mail and correspondence; identifying coins and paper money; making change; telling time; and using talking devices (e.g., clocks, watches, timers, calculators, digital organizers, memo recorders, audio labels).

A sample procedure for identifying coins and bills follows:

- Coins may be identified by size, thickness, and texture (e.g., milled or smooth edges). The dime and penny differ in size, and the quarter is larger than the nickel. The dime and quarter are milled around the edge; the nickel and penny are smooth.
- Bills can be folded for identification to different lengths and arranged in a definite (and consistent) pattern in the compartments of the billfold or wallet. A sighted individual must identify or confirm the bill denomination the first time it is used. A "talking" (voice output) bill identifier can be useful, but it is quite costly.
- Because the dollar bill is most often used, it should be left unfolded and can be placed as is, in the front of the wallet.
- The 5-dollar bill is folded in half so that it is the same height as the dollar bills when placed in the wallet. It goes in the same section as the dollar bills, on the right side of the compartment, with the folded edge up.
- The 10-dollar bill is folded twice and placed, folded edge up, on the left side of the bill compartment.
- The 20-dollar bill is folded the same way as the 10 but is placed in the back compartment on the right side; or some people prefer to fold them once, horizontally, so that they are easily distinguished.

Selection and Use of Nonoptical Assistive Devices

A number of studies have documented that the proper use of devices, techniques, and training methods can successfully maximize the use of remaining vision in persons with low vision. Training in the use of magnification, illumination, and contrast, along with environmental modifications, has been found to be effective. (Goodrich & Mehr, 1986, p. 121)

To provide the most comprehensive training, occupational therapists must become familiar with low vision and other assistive devices to enhance the use of residual vision or to compensate for lack of vision. A sample list follows, but it does not begin to enumerate all of the available devices.

- *Self-care devices:* talking glucose monitors, insulin injection aids, medication organizers, eyedrop guides, talking thermometers, talking scales, magnifiers, high-magnification makeup mirrors, shaving systems, dressing aids.
- *Eating and drinking devices:* liquid-level indicators, sectioned or high-side dishes, food bumpers, adapted utensils.
- *Cooking and food preparation devices:* tactile or talking microwaves, tactually marked toasters or broiler ovens, temperature control cookware, beverage makers, adapted food processors and blenders, pan and pot holders, oven mitts, cool handles, measuring devices, cutting devices, knife guides, tongs, heat diffusers, adapted peelers and slicers.
- *Domestic tasks:* adapted switches, wall plates, tactual thermostats, reachers, needle threaders and other sewing devices, ironing guides, laundry devices.
- *Communications:* adapted or talking television remotes; key-finding devices; writing and signature guides; coin and key holders; low vision, talking, braille, and large-print watches, clocks, and timers; adapted and variable-speed recording devices; location finders; adapted or bold-tip markers and pens; labeling devices; clothing identifiers; book rests and holders; voice print speakers; adapted or large-print telephones and amplifiers.

Creating Safe and Functional Environments for People With Low Vision

Making a private or public environment safe and functional for people who are blind or visually impaired should be part of universal design that will benefit all users of a facility, whether it is a workplace, museum, a senior center, or a home. Making facilities, programs, and activities safe and accessible for older participants with visual impairments does not necessarily require a great deal of time, energy, or money. It is a matter of understanding the basic elements, and planning for easy access during the initial design and layout, or in adapting the environment, as needed.

The use of lighting and color contrast, and the reduction of glare, are the basic elements to consider. The suggestions that follow can be used to conduct an assessment of the environment. A vision rehabilitation professional can provide further assistance in assessing the environment and making recommendations for changes to enhance safe and independent functioning and active participation in daily living routines.

Environmental Adaptations or Modifications and Lighting

Usually the challenge in providing adequate lighting is to provide optimal illumination without producing glare. Methods of increasing light on a task include bringing the light closer to the task, adding more lights, and changing the background of the task so that contrast is increased. For example, using a solid white or light-colored place mat under a dark mug or dish. (Watson & Berg, 1983, p. 343)

When people have difficulty seeing, they will often become frustrated and inefficient in the performance of daily tasks. Improved lighting, both quality and quantity of light, should help. Correct lighting is probably the most important nonoptical visual aid both for people with normal vision and for those with impaired vision. However, increased quantity of light alone may do little to help a person with low vision to see an object (or words on a page) if there is glare or insufficient color and shading contrast between the object and the background. Often, increasing the wattage of incandescent bulbs increases glare (Carter, 1983).

Therefore, simply increasing the wattage of a bulb may not be the best solution. Moreover, a person can have the most accommodating lenses and lighting for the purpose of reading, but if the desk or table on which the book rests has a color value the same as the written page, neither glasses nor magnifiers or other optical devices will help the person see better. However, a desk that is simply darker in color than the page would be a tremendous help. Any improvements in lighting, color, or contrast must be practical, simple, and economical.

Types of Light

Five kinds of lights are appropriate for various activities and functions: (a) sunlight/ natural, (b) incandescent (standard light bulbs), (c) fluorescent (tubes or bulbs), (d) combination incandescent and fluorescent, and (e) halogen.

Natural light is ideal for most everyday tasks, but it is inconsistent throughout the day. Natural light also tends to cause dangerous shadows and glare.

Incandescent light is concentrated and not preferred for general room lighting because, like sunlight, it tends to create shadows. As wattage increases, the lights produce more heat. Full-spectrum incandescent bulbs are closest to natural sunlight and produce the brightest illumination.

Fluorescent light is most commonly used in office, school, and clinic settings. It can be "warm" or "cool" light, depending on the bulb. It illuminates a wider area than incandescent light and does not create shadows. However, because fluorescent light is commonly ceiling installed, the light produced is more diffuse and less focused on a task at table height. The newest type of fluorescent lights, called *compact fluorescent lamps,* fit into regular lamp sockets. They provide illumination comparable to incandescent light but produce less heat and use less energy.

Combination light uses both incandescent and fluorescent bulbs and is the most functional and comfortable light for everyday activities. This type of light most closely approximates natural sunlight. You can devise this type of lighting by using the two types of bulbs in a current fixture with two sockets.

Halogen light is sometimes preferred because it is more focused, brighter, whiter, and more concentrated and energy efficient than incandescent light. However, because halogen light is hotter, it is more intense, and it requires a protective shield. It is not recommended for prolonged close work. Halogen light should be used with caution as it produces intense heat and can cause severe burns and personal injury if used incorrectly. This is especially true for people with low vision who may reach for the fixture or lamp in a way that is dangerous.

General Recommendations for Lighting

The following four recommendations may help low vision adults:

1. In recreation and reading areas, provide ample floor and table lamps.
2. Advise people with visual impairments that light should always be aimed at the task they are doing, not at their eyes (*task lighting*).
3. Replace burned out light bulbs regularly.
4. Place mirrors so that lighting does not reflect off them and create glare.
   - For window coverings, use adjustable blinds, sheer curtains, or draperies because they allow for the adjustment of natural light.
   - Place a chair near (but not facing) a window for reading or doing handcrafts near natural light.
   - Strongly discourage removal of covers or shades from lamps or light fixtures. Bare bulbs cause extreme glare, eye fatigue, dangerous shadows, and possible "blind spots" for anyone in the environment.

Recommendations for the Kitchen

The kitchen is notorious for its lack of color contrast. Walls, ceilings, sinks, refrigerators, cupboards, and counters are usually a light color and provide little or no background contrast for light-colored objects, liquids, and foods. Therefore, people with low vision have great difficulty in measuring quantities, portioning foods into desired amounts, reading gauges, judging cooking time, and addressing physical hazards and safety. The following suggestions can help:

- To the wall area above a kitchen counter, attach a sheet of dark-colored contact paper. If the existing wall is brightly colored, apply a sheet of white contact paper to create contrast for pouring dark- or light-colored liquid or for measuring or cutting foods.
- In the dining area, recommend light-colored dinnerware on a dark table or tablecloth, or the reverse. Avoid patterned placemats, tablecloths, or dinnerware, as they tend to confuse the eye. The simplicity of solid, high-contrast colors is best.
- Although it is difficult in the kitchen, use incandescent lighting instead of (or in addition to) fluorescent, whenever possible. Avoid very bright, unshaded illumination from overhead light sources that can cast heavy shadows. If at all possible place the light source below or at eye level . A swing-arm table lamp on the kitchen counter is ideal.

Recommendations for the Bathroom

Lighting in the bathroom is probably more difficult and complicated than in any other area in the home. The most common lighting arrangement found in bathrooms is the wall light fixture located above the mirrored medicine cabinet. This provides an illuminated, reflected image for grooming. The higher above eye level the light fixture is located, the worse it is for the person with low vision, because it deepens the shadows of facial features. This can be disastrous for shaving, applying makeup, or inserting eyedrops.

An alternate lighting arrangement is the mirrored medicine cabinet with built-in fluorescent fixtures on either side. This illuminates the face more uniformly and eliminates facial shadows. Placing light fixtures lower will always improve the ability to use residual vision. Another possibility is to install adjustable swing-arm lamps wherever additional flexible lighting is needed for personal grooming. As in the kitchen, the tendency in the bathroom runs toward light-colored walls, ceilings, and tile flooring, lacking any significant contrast. Applying contact paper for contrast near the mirror, or painting a dark border around the medicine cabinet, can be helpful. To reduce glare, always use low-gloss or flat-finish paint or wall covering.

Recommendations for the Living Area

Use scattered light sources throughout the room rather than overhead lighting of any kind, or combine these sources of light. Use desk and floor lamps with adjustable arms, if possible, to specifically direct illumination for reading. Install dimmer switches to reduce glare by increasing or decreasing light levels in relationship to the task or activity (i.e., brighter for reading, dimmer for watching television). Shield light sources, such as windows, from direct view. The use of dimmer switches for room lighting, and three-way bulbs in lamps, provides more flexibility as lighting needs change throughout the day.

A dark, open-weave drape or adjustable blind will significantly reduce the sun's glare and add contrast to its surroundings. Modify surfaces that are shiny or glass topped to reduce reflection. One of the most common misconceptions among older people is that "brighter is better," so they tend to use bare bulbs without shades; however, as mentioned earlier in the general recommendations, the glare makes it extremely difficult to use residual vision in an optimal way.

If there are laundry facilities in the home, install adjustable swing-arm lighting over the washing machine and dryer and suggest a hand-held magnifier for reading the washer and dryer controls.

Modifications or Adaptations of the Overall Environment

It is important to remember that vision and visual needs may fluctuate dramatically during periods of the day, or from day to day (Sicurella, 1977). One must respect the concerns of an individual with regard to aesthetics and familiarity in the placement of objects and furnishings in the home. Both RTs and occupational therapists might recommend the following adaptations or modifications:

- Leave furniture and personal items in the same location once they have been positioned safely. This helps orient the person with low vision to the environment and reduces tripping accidents and falls. Advise family members, caregivers, housekeepers, and maintenance personnel not to move furniture or personal items without informing the person with low vision. Even the slightest repositioning can be totally disorienting. This is one of the most common complaints made by people with low vision.

- Keep the largest pieces of furniture against walls and out of the path of circulation, if possible. Make sure that no furniture that is low to the ground (e.g., coffee tables) causes an obstruction in the path of movement. These objects present a serious hazard, especially to individuals who have lost peripheral vision in the lower segment of the visual field. The lower the object, the greater the possibility of tripping over it. When purchasing new furniture, select upholstery with texture when possible. Texture provides tactile clues for identification.

- Avoid hanging or protruding objects (e.g., hanging plants) at head or eye level. These objects present a serious hazard for individuals who have lost peripheral vision in the upper segment of the visual field, or who have lost central vision.

- Instruct persons with low vision and their families to keep all doors and cabinets either completely open or completely closed. Doors can be a major hazard if left ajar. Eliminate throw rugs, and check that all carpets and area rugs have skid-proof backing or are tacked to the floor. Loose carpeting on stairs can be especially hazardous.

- Consider purchasing a cordless telephone, which can be taken from room to room to enable the individual with low vision to answer the telephone without rushing for it.

- Mark edges of all steps and ramps with high-contrast paint or tape.

- In hallways, make sure that lighting is uniform throughout.

- If you mark or label an item in the home, such as stove dials, a microwave panel, or medication containers, make sure that everyone in the household can understand and use the marking system. Household members need to be advised not to move, eliminate, or modify the markings once they have been placed in the home.

- Whenever possible, plan any adaptations so that the person with low vision can maintain them over time independently (or with family assistance) with a minimum of effort.

- Paint doors and door frames in bright, solid colors that contrast with the wall color, to increase their visibility. Paint or purchase doorknobs or handles in a color that contrasts with that of the door. This will help people with low vision locate doors and exits quickly in case of an emergency. It will also help the person identify whether the door is open or closed.

- In the bathroom, place a contrasting-color, non-skid, textured bathmat in the shower or tub to prevent falls, and provide a cue for judging the depth of the tub water. Set or mark the faucet/controls on the hot water to a medium range temperature to reduce the danger of scalding.

Navigation and Wayfinding Techniques: The Sighted-Guide Technique

Orientation and mobility specialists and RTs focus on spatial relations and navigational techniques (e.g., trailing one's hand around the walls of a room to determine landmarks and location). Occupational therapists who work with people with low vision should, at the very least, be familiar with how to use and teach the *sighted-guide technique* (see Figure 6.1). It will be important to learn this technique so that one can teach it to the person with low vision as well as to other staff members. Occupational therapists should consult with vision rehabilitation professionals for complete in-service training in this area.

The purpose of the sighted-guide technique is to enable an individual with low vision to travel safely and efficiently with a sighted person in unfamiliar environments and under varying conditions.

Grasp and Position

- The person with low vision should grasp the sighted guide's arm just above the elbow, with his or her fingers on the inside and thumb on the outside.
- The person with low vision then keeps his or her upper arm vertical (tucked in) at the side, with the forearm flexed at approximately 90°, or parallel with the ground.
- The person with low vision is now positioned a half-step behind and to the side of the guide. The guide's arm remains tucked in, as well, and also at 90°.
- If the guide has an unusually large arm, or is exceptionally tall, or there is a drastic difference in height between the two, the person with low vision can grasp the guide's forearm or wrist. This way, the guide's arm remains extended at his or her side, rather than flexed. When walking in a potentially dangerous or obstructed area (e.g., a cafeteria or crowded hallway), the person with low vision should be instructed to walk on the side furthest from the obstacles.

Adaptations to this technique can be made if the individual being guided has an upper-extremity limitation or disability such as arthritis, carpal tunnel syndrome, contractures, spasticity, tremors, or any other grasping/prehensile limitations.

General Suggestions for the Guide

- Make physical contact with the person with low vision by touching his or her arm before beginning to travel together.
- Briefly describe the environment and destination before beginning to travel.
- When you have arrived at your destination, make contact with some object or furnishing before leaving the person in an unfamiliar place, and indicate when you are leaving.

Narrow Passages and Doorways

- The guide moves his or her arm back, toward the center of his or her body, as a signal of a narrow passage, doorway, or changing terrain.

- The person being guided extends his or her arm, placing himself or herself one full step behind the guide. It is important to maintain this distance behind the guide so as not to step on the guide's heels. Because this particular technique offers more protection than the regular sighted-guide technique, it also may be used when the person being guided is uncertain of his or her footing or of the pace of travel.

Closed Doors

- The guide pauses before a door, alerting the individual being guided.
- If the doorway is narrow, the person being guided follows a full step behind the guide.
- The guide must indicate to which side the door will open (toward or away from them), whether the door is particularly heavy, and whether it is self-closing.

Stairs

- The guide should indicate that stairs are being approached and whether they ascend or descend. The guide should momentarily pause at the landing and instruct the person to locate the stair edge with his or her foot.
- The guide proceeds up or down one step ahead of the person. The guide's upward or downward movement indicates that ascent or descent has begun.
- The guide should pause momentarily on the last step to indicate the approach of the landing.
- If available, a railing should always be used. The guide places the person's hand on the railing to indicate location and direction (ascending or descending).
- If there are two or more flights of stairs, the guide makes square corners (90° turns) when traveling from one flight to another.

Chair Seating

The guide should place the person in contact with some part of the chair and allow the person to seat himself or herself as follows:

- Place the person's hand on the back of the chair first, and follow down the back to the seat of the chair.
- Have the person make a half circle on the seat with his or her hand to make sure the chair is empty and usable. Before the person sits down, have him or her turn around so that the backs of the knees or legs touch the seat of the chair. Allow the person to reach for armrests, if they exist, and then sit down while maintaining contact with the chair.

Psychosocial Aspects of Low Vision and Related Issues

The impact of blindness is that many people are left with a sense of abandonment. Feelings of discomfort result from asking family and friends for assistance. This discomfort frequently leads to avoidance. The person with a vision impairment wishing to avoid embarrassment learns not to "make demands," not to expose oneself to further hurt or rejection. Isolation and loneliness then become a part of the impact of vision loss (Freedman & Inkster, 1976, p. 13).

According to Father Carroll (author of *Blindness: What It Is, What It Does and How To Live With It;* 1961), a seminal writer who addressed the impact of vision loss in adults, the losses associated with sensory impairment include losses in psychological security, basic skills, communication, appreciation, occupation, and financial status, as well as a sense of wholeness.

It should not be difficult for professionals to understand the feelings of frustration and anxiety experienced from the impact of vision loss, especially when the condition is first discovered or acknowledged. Feelings of depression are appropriate and under-standable in grieving for the loss of one's sight and former lifestyle. The impact of such feelings should not be minimized in terms of their influence on learning capacity, reten-tion of information, and the ability to benefit from rehabilitation services.

Because it may be difficult for the therapist to deal with these very palpable reac-tions, sometimes the tendency is to avoid confronting or discussing them directly. Instead, attention is placed on training and skills that will facilitate independent func-tioning. By addressing the individual's reactions and feelings directly, and including these discussions as part of the rehabilitation process, the occupational therapist and other pro-fessionals will facilitate adjustment, particularly as new skills are learned that lead toward an increased feeling of competence and mastery.

Individuals may exhibit behaviors of such extreme magnitude, or with such self-destructive potential, that the therapist is alarmed or finds it difficult to initiate or con-tinue treatment. As in all situations involving extreme emotional impact and loss, refer-ral for a psychological evaluation or counseling is recommended. However, severe depres-sion requiring medication, or suicidal ideations, are not the typical behavior of a person with vision loss. It is more likely that the therapist will observe behaviors that range from sadness and anger to withdrawal, self-consciousness, and helplessness.

In addition to the impact of emotional and economic losses experienced by the per-son with low vision, relationships with family, friends, and the general community are altered. The need to ask for assistance can drastically change a person's self-perception, self-image, and sense of self-worth. For instance, asking for help in reading correspon-dence highlights the person's awareness of the loss both of reading ability and of privacy.

No one adjusts to change, to loss, or to impairment in a vacuum, or entirely independently. The success or failure of adjustment, and certainly the rate of adjustment, depends on individual coping strategies and the involvement and reactions of significant others. (Orr, 1991, p. 7)

"While the older visually impaired person's primary goal is to continue to be as indepen-dent as possible, of equal value is the ability to be interdependent with the family and within the social context" (Orr, 1991, p. 9).

This theoretical discussion is brought to life in direct conversation with people who experience vision loss:

> What have these elders told us of the experience of vision loss that extends beyond the particularities of their individual situations ? First, loss of vision in old age is no small thing. It permeates all aspects of life. And it hurts a lot: anxiety, frustration, aggravation, caution, fear and grief are frequent accompaniments. Time is not necessarily a healer. Due to changing life circumstances and the progressive nature of most vision impairments, attitude change may just as likely be for the worse as for the better. . . . Elders look both from within and outside for support. Medical attention is important, but it is recognized that it is not the only answer. Patience, doing what one can for oneself, keeping active, prayer, humor and tears may also help. (Burack-Weiss, 1991, p. 23)

An Example of a State Agency Serving People Who Are Blind or Have Low Vision

In New York State, the Commission for the Blind and Visually Handicapped (CBVH) has been responsible since 1913 for the coordination, oversight, quality assurance, and state funding for services for people of all ages who are legally blind. The commission contracts with 17 not-for-profit vision rehabilitation agencies in the state, as well as independent living centers and other providers. CBVH is a department within the New York State Office of Children and Family Services.

People with substantial vision loss but who are not legally blind are served through a different state department, called Vocational and Educational Services for People with Disabilities (VESID), which is part of the New York State Department of Education. VESID is exclusively a vocational entity, with no services for children and senior citizens.

In 1984, New York State passed legislation with a state appropriation to expand services for children and senior citizens who are blind through CBVH. The programs for senior citizens were based on client-determined goals and outcomes, a "consumer-driven rehabilitation plan." The success of this model and its several iterations solidified the commitment of CBVH to fund services for blind senior citizens.

Currently in New York State, the updated program is called the Adaptive Living Program (ALP), and it serves blind persons ages 54 and older. ALP services reach approximately 4,000 legally blind people each year.

If you are interested in finding services in your area, or how to access vision rehabilitation in your state, the following are some suggestions:

- Search the Directory of Services published on CD-ROM or the AFB Web site.
- Search your state government Web site for the local entity or department that serves people who are blind or low vision.
- Contact the federal Rehabilitation Services Administration regional office covering your area, the U.S. Department of Veterans Affairs, or the local Veterans

Administration Hospital, all of which can be located through the government pages of your local telephone directory.

- Contact the American Academy of Ophthalmology or the American Optometric Association (see Appendix 6.A).

Role of a Not-for-Profit Vision Rehabilitation Agency in the Provision of Services

About VISIONS: A Multidisciplinary Service Setting

Before 1970, vision rehabilitation and social services were not readily available for senior citizens who are blind or have low vision. Public and private funds were earmarked for those who were young and vocationally oriented. Owing to this lack of financial support, little was done nationally to develop programs to meet the multifaceted needs of senior citizens with low vision. VISIONS/Services for the Blind and Visually Impaired, however, was a leader in the 1960s and 1970s in the development of vision rehabilitation, recreation, volunteer, senior center mainstream activities, and community education programs for senior citizens with low vision.

Many vision rehabilitation agencies operate hotlines or information-and-referral centers. The call center in New York State is a database search service called "Blindline sm (service mark)" and is housed at VISIONS; it is staffed by a director and interns who are legally blind. Recreation services are frequently part of the service mix. VISIONS sponsors Vacation Camp for the Blind in Rockland County, New York, which provides year-round rehabilitation, therapeutic recreation, and social services for people who are blind or visually impaired, all ages. VISIONS at Selis Manor is a community center in New York City for blind adults and senior citizens; it offers vision rehabilitation, counseling, and self-development and education classes.

Vision rehabilitation agencies offer specialized services and train local community providers to offer their services in a way that is more sensitive and welcoming for people with vision loss. VISIONS helps local senior centers make their activities accessible and trains case managers in local agencies to identify and refer people with vision loss for vision rehabilitation services.

The VISIONS rehabilitation service model is primarily home and community based. Service plans are individualized and are based on the person's expressed and demonstrated needs. The goal of this model includes skills training to promote independence as well as use of and equal access to community services and resources. Since 1981, VISIONS has employed a full-time occupational therapist as part of the multidisciplinary vision rehabilitation team. VISIONS programs are funded by a mix of government, foundation, private, and investment dollars.

Case Example

The following case example describes an adventitiously blind adult's experience with vision rehabilitation services.

Jane (a pseudonym) is a 76-year-old widow living alone at home. She has no home care or family. She has a medical and eye history of glaucoma and cataracts, spinal stenosis, and osteoarthritis, and recently had a cardiovascular accident (CVA) with mild residual left hemiplegia. She is ambulatory with the use of a quadruped cane, and she exhibits some lower-extremity weakness and poor standing balance but no paralysis. Her left upper extremity exhibits mild spasticity with limited range of motion, poor coordination, and some evidence of neuropathy in the left hand. Jane is independent in self-care skills.

She reads large print with the use of a magnifier, but her vision fluctuates from day to day, and she reports only seeing a "blur" at times. She has difficulty seeing faces, and her depth perception is compromised. She was introduced to the agency when the social worker from her HMO clinic contacted the Commission for the Blind, and she was referred for services. The social worker called on Jane's behalf because Jane had been diagnosed as legally blind by her ophthalmologist and was reporting difficulty completing household chores and traveling in the community.

Although instruction in these ADL had been provided through traditional medical rehabilitation services following her stroke, Jane had made few gains. After a lengthy interview with an intake worker, an RT was assigned to work with Jane on a weekly basis. Through the use of adaptive techniques and nonoptical adaptive equipment introduced by the RT, Jane's home became increasingly more accessible to her. Raised dots (tactual markings) placed on the stove dials, oven, and microwave enabled her to more easily and safely identify temperature settings, reheat food in the microwave, and regulate the flame on the stovetop burners, so she no longer burned herself when preparing meals.

At the same time, she was referred to a low vision optometrist. The low vision evaluation included a thorough eye examination, testing of acuity, measurement of eye pressure, cataract status, measurement of visual fields, refraction, and the introduction of various lenses to determine which ones allowed her to see more clearly. After testing a variety of optical aids and devices lent to her for home practice, Jane returned to the low vision doctor for a follow-up visit to select the best devices and for further training in the use of the newly prescribed equipment. She ultimately began to use a high-magnification screen enlarger to watch television, a hand-held monocular telescope to identify street signs when traveling outdoors, a high-powered stand magnifier for reading mail, and a folding pocket magnifier for use when shopping. She was given Noir UV glasses for outdoors (providing 100% UV and glare protection) and a halogen floor lamp with an adjustable arm, height adjustment, and weighted base for task lighting.

An O&M specialist evaluated Jane for independent travel both indoors and outdoors. With Jane's approval, the specialist began by covering Jane's quad cane in red and white reflective tape, to identify her as a person with low vision. However, during their respective evaluations, both the RT and O&M specialist observed difficulties in completion of tasks, as well as functional deficits in orientation/reorientation, balance, retention of information, and transfers. An occupational therapist was asked to conduct a thorough assessment before continuing other services.

The occupational therapist began her participation in the team process by conducting an in-home evaluation. She observed that Jane exhibited difficulty in positioning, spatial awareness, and performance of ADL. Jane's inability to freely position her upper extremities (her left shoulder flexion was limited to 40°) for protective techniques within her own home was noted. In addition, she exhibited poor spatial and environmental concept development; compromised ADL skills requiring motor planning and sequencing of steps (e.g., meal preparation); visual field deficits and directionality limitations necessary for learning fine motor tasks such as simple sewing or total body involvement in such activities as bed-making. Some spasticity and left-upper-extremity weakness, with limitations in dexterity and coordination, were evident. In communications skills, Jane was unable to print her name, not only because she had difficulty seeing the page but also because she could not consistently find the left side of the paper. She could not move the pen in the proper direction or identify reference points on the page, because of hemianopsia and left-side neglect.

Jane was found to have difficulty in isolating body parts for purposeful movement, and in laterally flexing her neck or trunk, because of spinal stenosis due to the residual effects of the CVA. Proprioception, spatial awareness, and body concepts were below average.

Transfers in bathing and toileting were observed. Because of vestibular and visual deficits, a high-color-contrast grab bar and bathtub mat were installed in the shower, a bath seat was installed and fitted with a piece of contrasting color dycem mat, and extensive training in transfer safety techniques was provided. Tasks requiring simultaneous movements were incorporated into her treatment plan, along with various motor planning activities as an enhancement to RT training. The latter began as very simple bilateral tasks and later included reciprocal patterns and more complex bilateral skills.

One-to-one occupational therapy sessions included specific prehensile tasks to improve dexterity and coordination and introduction of signature and letter-writing guides and their placement to help her compensate for her left-side neglect. Jane exhibited mild dressing apraxia and difficulty sequencing, although she was able to dress independently. Her eating skills were intact, although she tended to ignore food and utensils on the left side of her plate.

Visual scanning techniques were applied to improve her eating skills and reclaim her self-confidence in going to restaurants.

The occupational therapist and RT worked collaboratively with Jane on specific bilateral activities such as boiling water, pouring liquids safely, reheating food in the microwave, measuring amounts, cutting and peeling, and using the stovetop burners. In addition, sequencing her dressing process, as well as organizing her clothes and accessories, and using braille tags for identification, allowed her to be more independent and self-confident.

Jane's writing became legible when she learned to use adapted writing, check, and signature guides. In addition, she learned a portion of the braille alphabet, which she used primarily for marking labels for clothing, medicine containers, spice and condiment jars, and other household items. Instruction in the use of a large-print/talking calculator helped Jane manage her finances and checkbook independently.

As treatment progressed, she developed increased fluidity of movement, improved balance and coordination, all of which was a prerequisite for further O&M instruction. Jane also significantly improved her ability to sequence tasks and was able to apply this skill to the use of a long cane and quad cane simultaneously for outdoor travel, on days when her vision was severely diminished. In general, in occupational therapy, RT, and O&M, she learned complicated tasks with greater ease, suggesting improved motor planning.

An opportunity for recreation and social activities was offered to Jane, who was encouraged to join a nearby senior center. The staff at the center received an in-service in adaptive techniques from an occupational therapist and sensitivity training to further ensure the incorporation of other visually impaired senior citizens into their program. The occupational therapist also conducted an informal environmental survey of the senior center at the request of the director, for accessibility, lighting and glare, color contrast, signage, and safety. Environmental modifications were recommended to make the facility more user friendly for Jane and other people with visual impairments.

The O&M specialist conducted mobility lessons outdoors to enable Jane to walk the three blocks to the center with a long cane or, when needed, with both the quad and long canes simultaneously. Because of her upper-extremity spasticity, neuropathy, and weakness, this presented a challenge, but Jane persevered. The O&M specialist also addressed Jane's safety in navigating the center once she arrived. Jane now attends the center several times weekly, and she has developed many new friendships there.

Jane was also given information and assistance in applying for a summer camp for the blind in Spring Valley, New York, which she attended the following summer.

Conclusion

Objectives and accurate measures of the effects of treatment need to be more extensively applied to the functional performance of people with low vision. Beginning efforts to measure outcomes do exist.

When approaching a person with vision loss, it is important to realize that there are no unarguable rules that fit or apply to everyone. No two people have the same type or degree of vision loss; lifestyle; home environment; or needs, desires, or preferences. In this chapter we have addressed the spectrum of vision loss, surveyed the field of vision rehabilitation, and offered techniques and therapeutic solutions for treating adults with visual impairments. Some techniques are borrowed from the wisdom and expertise of vision rehabilitation professionals. Some are inherent in the current occupational therapy paradigm that addresses the treatment of all aspects of the life of a person with a disability. Rehabilitation for people with low vision or who are blind offers occupational therapists an opportunity to exercise their wide range of talents, from activity analysis to psychosocial adjustment, while incorporating the specialized knowledge base from the field of vision rehabilitation.

The ideal location for training is the person's own home or residence. Rehabilitation goals become more relevant to the needs of the individual on a day-to-day basis if they are established and taught in a familiar setting. For an occupational therapist who is primarily a clinical practitioner, it must be recognized that the person with low vision may have difficulty transferring techniques and adaptations for independent living to their everyday reality at home.

The nature of vision loss, with its frequent result of isolation and social withdrawal, translates into lack of access or involvement in the very services that could prevent isolation, increase independence, and improve quality of life. Outreach to all people who can benefit from vision rehabilitation and the provision of services to those in need, especially elderly people, remain unmet goals.

Occupational therapists, by the nature of their training, use positive energy and reinforcement to help people help themselves and maintain the center of control of their lives. They are problem solvers and facilitators and, therefore, are a critical resource for people with visual impairments. However, to provide these services, specialized vision rehabilitation techniques and experience are required. In addition, knowledge of ocular pathology, optics, functional use of magnification, low vision evaluation protocols, and adaptive devices specific to low vision must be developed.

Finally, collaboration with colleagues in the field of rehabilitation in the traditional vision service network is essential. Occupational therapists will then be in a position to apply their unique expertise and expand the likelihood of positive outcomes for the growing numbers of people with low vision or who are blind.

References

American Foundation for the Blind. (1972). *An introduction to working with the aging person who is visually handicapped.* New York: Author.

American Foundation for the Blind. (1999). *Talking points on Title VII, Chapter 2 for personal visits.* New York: Author.

American Foundation for the Blind. (2000). *Statistics and sources for professionals: Prevalence.* New York: Author.

American Occupational Therapy Association. (2001). *Occupational therapy practice guidelines for adults with low vision.* Bethesda, MD: Author.

Anderson, D. R. (1982). *Testing the field of vision.* St. Louis, MO: Mosby.

Balanced Budget Refinement Act of 1999, Pub. L, 106–113.

Branch, L., Horowitz, A., & Carr, C. (1989). The implication for everyday life of the incidence of self-reported visual decline among people over age 65 living in the community. *The Gerontologist, 29,* 359–365.

Burack-Weiss, A. (1991). In their own words: Elders' reactions to vision loss. In N. Weber (Ed.), *Vision and aging: Issues in social work practice* (pp. 15–23). Binghamton, NY: Haworth Press.

Carroll, T. (1961). *Blindness: What it is, what it does, and how to live with it.* Boston: Little, Brown.

Carter, K. (1983). Assessment of lighting. In R. Jose (Ed.), *Understanding low vision* (pp. 403–414). New York: American Foundation for the Blind.

Centers for Medicare and Medicaid Services. (2002, May 29). Program Memorandum Transmittal AB-02-078, Department of Health and Human services (DHHS). Washington, DC: Author.

Duane, T. D. (Ed.). (1990). *Clinical ophthalmology.* New York: Harper & Row.

Duffy, M. (2002). *Making life more livable: Simple adaptations for living at home after vision loss* (rev. ed.). New York: American Foundation for the Blind.

Faye, E. (1984). *Clinical low vision* (2nd ed.). Boston: Little, Brown.

Fox, C., & Kern, T. (1992). *Understanding low vision rehabilitation and the implications for occupational therapy.* Bethesda, MD: American Occupational Therapy Association.

Freedman, S., & Inkster, D. (1976). *The impact of blindness in the aging process.* New York: VISIONS/Services for the Blind and Visually Impaired.

Gentile, M. (Ed.). (1997). *Functional visual behavior: A therapist's guide to evaluation and treatment options.* Bethesda, MD: American Occupational Therapy Association.

Goodrich, G., & Mehr, E. (1986). Eccentric viewing training and low vision aids. *American Journal of Optometry and Physiological Optics, 63,* 119–126.

Kern, T. (1996). Viewpoints on working with people with low vision. *OT Practice, 1,* 19.

Kern, T., & Weiss, D. (2000). *A diagram: Distinct and shared aspects between OT and O&M/RT.* New York: VISIONS.

Lampert, J., & Lapolice, D. (1995). Functional considerations in evaluation and treatment of the client with low vision. *American Journal of Occupational Therapy, 49,* 885.

Orr, A. (1991). The psychosocial aspects of aging and vision loss. In N. Weber (Ed.), *Vision and aging: Issues in social work practice* (pp. 1–14). Binghamton, NY: Haworth Press.

Orr, A. (Ed.). (1992). *Vision and aging: Crossroads for service delivery.* New York: American Foundation for the Blind.

Orr, A., & Rogers, P. (2002). *Solutions for everyday living for older people with visual impairment.* New York: American Foundation for the Blind.

Phillips, T., & Correia, A., (1979). Internal document. New York: Center for Independent Living, New York.

Rehabilitation Act of 1973, Pub. L, 93–112, 29 U.S.C. § 701 *et seq.*

Rehabilitation Act of 1973 Amendments, Pub. L, 95–602, H.R. 12467, H. Rept. 95-1149.

Ringgold, N. P. (1991). *Out of the corner of my eye: Living with vision loss in later life.* New York: American Foundation for the Blind.

Rogers, J. C. (1981). Gerontic occupational therapy. *American Journal of Occupational Therapy, 35,* 663–666.

Sicurella, V. (1977). Color contrast as an aid for visually impaired persons. *Journal of Visual Impairment and Blindness, 71,* 252–257.

VISIONS/Services for the Blind and Visually Impaired. (2000). *Purpose and role of occupational therapy at VISIONS/Services for the Blind and Visually Impaired.* Unpublished report.

Warren, M. (1995). Including occupational therapy in low vision rehabilitation. *American Journal of Occupational Therapy, 49,* 857–860.

Warren, M. (2000) *Low vision: Occupational therapy intervention with the older adult.* Bethesda MD: Occupational Therapy Association.

Watson, G., & Berg, R. (1983). Near training techniques. In R. Jose (Ed.), *Understanding low vision* (pp. 317–362). New York: American Foundation for the Blind.

Woosley, T., Harden, R., & Murphy, P. (1983). *SPOTR: Screening for Physical and Occupational Therapy Referral.* Talladega: Alabama Institute for Deaf Blind.

Zuckerman, D. M. (2004). *Blind adults in America: Their lives and challenges.* Washington, DC: National Center for Policy Research for Women and Families.

Selected Readings

Bachelder, J., & Harkins, D. (1995). Do occupational therapists have a primary role in low vision rehabilitation? *American Journal of Occupational Therapy, 49,* 927–930.

Baker-Nobles, L., & Bink, M. (1979). Sensory integration in the rehabilitation of blind adults. *American Journal of Occupational Therapy, 33,* 559–564.

Boone, S., Watson, D., & Bagley, M. (1994). *The challenge to independence: Vision and hearing loss among older adults.* Little Rock: University of Arkansas Rehabilitation Research Training Center.

Dickman, I. (1983). *Making life more livable: Simple adaptations for the homes of blind and visually impaired older people.* New York: American Foundation for the Blind.

Duane, T. D. (Ed.). (1981–1990). *Clinical ophthalmology.* New York: Harper & Row.

Duffy, M., & Beliveau-Tobey, M. (Eds.). (1991). *New independence for older persons with vision loss in long-term care facilities.* New York: AWARE.

Fletcher, D. C., Shindell, S., Hindman, T., & Schaffrath, M. (1991). Low vision rehabilitation: Finding capable people behind damaged eyeballs. *Western Journal of Medicine, 154,* 554–556.

Fox, C. (1993). Visual and vestibular function. In H. Cohen (Ed.), *Neuroscience for rehabilitation.* (pp. 97–128). Philadelphia: Lippincott.

Hazekamp, J., & Lundin, J. (Eds.). (1986). *Program guidelines for visually impaired individuals.* Sacramento, CA: State Department of Education.

Ingalls, J. (1972). *A trainer's guide to andragogy: Its concepts, experience and application.* Washington, DC: U.S. Department of Health, Education, and Welfare.

Kern, T., & Shaw, C. (1985). *An interdisciplinary approach to training the adult blind client.* New York: VISIONS/Services for the Blind and Visually Impaired.

Lampert, J. (1994). Occupational therapists, O&M specialists, and rehabilitation teachers. *Journal of Visual Impairment and Blindness, 88,* 297–298.

The Lighthouse. (1995). *National survey on vision loss.* New York: Author.

Ludwig, I., & Schneider, P. (1991). A model of comprehensive community-based services for older blind adults. In N. Weber (Ed.), *Vision and aging: Issues in social work practice* (pp. 25–36). Binghamton, NY: Haworth Press.

Mulholland, M. (Ed.). (1993). Diabetes [Special issue]. *Journal of Visual Impairment and Blindness, 87.*

Orr, A., & Heubner, K. (2001). Toward a collaborative working relationship among vision rehabilitation and allied professionals. *Journal of Visual Impairment and Blindness, 95,* 468–482.

Rosenbloom, A., & Morgan, M. (Eds.). (1986). *Vision and aging: General and clinical perspectives.* New York: Professional Press Books/Fairchild.

Ruben, B. (1990, June 28). A new vision: OT brings insight to the field of visual impairment. *OT Week, 4,* pp. 4–5.

Wainapel, S. (1989). Severe visual impairment on a rehabilitation unit: Incidence and implications. *Archives of Physical Medicine and Rehabilitation, 70,* 439–441.

Warren, M., & Lampert, J. (1994). Considerations in addressing the daily living needs in older persons with low vision. In A. Colenbrander & D. C. Fletcher (Eds.), *Low vision and vision rehabilitation: Ophthalmology Clinics of North America, 7,* 194.

Warren, M. (Ed.). (1995). Low vision [Special issue]. *American Journal of Occupational Therapy, 49,* 857–860.

Weber, N. (Ed.). (1991). *Vision and aging: Issues in social work practice.* Binghamton, NY: Haworth Press.

Williams, H., Webb, A., & Phillips, W. (1993). *Outcome funding: A new approach to targeted grant-making* (2nd ed.). New York: Rensselaerville Institute.

Yeadon, A. (1978). *Toward independence: The use of instructional objectives in teaching daily living skills to the blind.* New York: American Foundation for the Blind.

Appendix 6.A
Resources

- **Academy for the Certification of Vision Rehabilitation and Education Professionals,** 330 N. Commerce Park Loop, No. 200, Tucson, AZ 85745; 520-887-6816.

- **American Academy of Ophthalmology,** PO Box 7424, San Francisco, CA 94120; 415-561-8555, ext. 223; http://www.eyenet.org.

- **American Foundation for the Blind,** 11 Penn Plaza, Suite 300, New York, NY 10001; 212-502-7600; 800-232-5463; http://www.aft.org.
  Maintains national directory of services, reference library, information services, National Technology Center, latest computer adaptations, and scholarships and grants for people in need.

- **American Occupational Therapy Association,** 4720 Montgomery Lane, Bethesda, MD 20814; 800-729-2682; www.aota.org.

- **American Optometric Association,** 243 N. Lindbergh Boulevard, St. Louis, MO 63141; 800-365-2219; www.aota.org.

- **Association for Education and Rehabilitation of the Blind and Visually Impaired,** 1703 N. Beauregard Street, Suite 440, Alexandria, VA 22311-1744; 877-492-2708; aernet@laser.net.
  Professional membership organization; conducts conferences, offers continuing education, publishes newsletter and journal; operates reference information center; certifies rehabilitation teachers, orientation and mobility specialists, and classroom teachers.

- **Association for the Education and Rehabilitation of the Blind and Visually Impaired,** *Re:View Rehabilitation and Education for Blindness and Visual Impairment.* Available from Heldref Publications, 1319 18th Street, NW, Washington, DC 20036; 800-365-9753; http://www.heldref.org.

- **Association for World Action in Rehabilitation and Education,** New Independence Publications, PO Box 96, Mohegan Lake, NY 10547; 914-528-0567; http://www.aware usa.org.
  Offers publications regarding low vision and educational materials and resources for visually impaired people.

- **BlindFam: Blindness and Family Life.**
  Discussions of all aspects of family life as they are affected by blindness in one or more family members. To subscribe to the e-mail newsletter, send this command in the body of an email: SUBSCRIBEBlindFam (your first name, last name) to listserv@sjuvm. bitnet. Free.

- **Blind Rehabilitation Services,** U.S. Department of Veterans Affairs, 810 Vermont Avenue, NW, Washington, DC 20420; 202-233-3232.
- **C Tech Catalog** (free), *Products for the Blind and Low Vision Community* (including closed-circuit televisions), c/o Chuck Cohen, PO Box 30, Pearl River, NY 10965; 914-735-7907, 800-228-7798.
- **Dazor Manufacturing Corporation,** 4483 Duncan Avenue, St. Louis, MO 63110; 800-345-9103.
  Largest manufacturer of adapted and magnified lighting. Free catalog.
- **Descriptive Video Service** (DVS), Home Video Catalog (free), c/o WGBH-TV, 125 Western Avenue, Boston, MA 02134.
  Describes movies for people with low (or no) vision. To listen to a demonstration of DVS using a touch-tone phone, hear listing of available titles, or request catalog, call 800-333-1203.
- **Doubleday Large Print Home Library,** 1225 S. Market Street, Mechanicsburg, PA 17055; http://www.doubledaylargeprint.com/.
- **Duffy, M., & Beliveau-Tobey, M. (Eds.). (1991).** *New independence for persons with vision loss in long-term care facilities. Volume 1: Facilitator guide. Volume 2: Learner workbook. Volume 3: Resource manual.* Available from AWARE, PO Box 96, Mohegan Lake, NY 10547; 914-528-0567; http://www.awareusa.org.
- **Glaucoma Research Foundation,** 490 Post Street, Suite 830, San Francisco, CA 94102; 415-986-3162.
- **Joint Commission on Allied Health Personnel in Opthalmology,** 2025 Woodlane Drive, St. Paul, MN 55125; 612-731-2944.
  Certifies low vision technicians, publishes *Outlook* and free newsletter.
- **Journal of Visual Impairment and Blindness,** American Foundation for the Blind Press, 11 Penn Plaza, Suite 300, New York, NY 10001; 800-232-3044; afbsub@abdintl.com; http://www.afb.org/store.
- **Keitzer Writing Guides,** K Enterprises, P.O. Box 1284, Lake Wales, FL 33853; 813-676-1805.
- **Library of Congress National Library Services for the Blind and Physically Handicapped,** 1291 Taylor Street, NW, Washington, DC 20542; 202-707-5100, 800-424-9100.
  Distributes free reading materials in braille and large print and on recorded cassettes.
- **Lighthouse International,** 111 E. 59th Street, New York, NY 10022; 800-829-0500; www.lighthouse.org. Free catalog.
- **Maxi Aids & Appliances for Independent Living,** PO Box 3209, Farmingdale, NY 11735; 800-522-6294; http://www.maxiaids.com.
  Offers products for blind, physically disabled, and hearing impaired people or senior citizens with special needs. Free catalog.
- **National Association for the Visually Handicapped,** 22 W. 21st Street, New York, NY 10010; 212-889-3141.
  Large-print reading material and advocacy for people with visual impairments.

- **National Center for Policy Research for Women and Families**, 1901 Pennsylvania Avenue, NW, Suite 901, Washington, DC 20006; 202-223-4000; http://www.center4 policy.org.
- **National Diabetes Information Clearinghouse**, PO Box NDIC, Bethesda, MD 20892.
- **National Eye Health Education Program**, 2020 Vision Place, Bethesda, MD 20892; 301-496-5248.
- **Prevent Blindness America**, 500 E. Remington Road, Schaumburg, IL 60173; 312-843-2020.
- **Recording for the Blind and Dyslexic**, 20 Roszel Road, Princeton, NJ 08540; 609-452-0606.
- **Screening for Physical and Occupational Therapy Referral**, National Independent Living Skills Project, Alabama Institute for Deaf and Blind, PO Box 698, 205 E. South Street, Talladega, AL 35150.
- **Telephone Services:** Contact your local phone company, ask for the Center for People with Disabilities. Available free of charge: large-print number overlay for rotary phones; large-print stick-on numbers for touch-tone phones; dial "0" overlay for push-button keypad, which dials the operator when any key is pressed; braille or large-print phone bills; free dial-operator privileges and directory assistance; adapted telephones with big buttons and volume control.
- **VISIONS**, 500 Greenwich Street, Third Floor, New York, NY 10013; 212-625-1616; www.cilpubs.com.
  VISIONS/Services for the Blind and Visually Impaired and the Center for Independent Living has a publications series, including self-study audiobooks (cassette tapes with large-print companion booklets), on the following topics: indoor mobility, personal management, and sensory development, and lesson plans on basic indoor mobility, personal management, and sensory development.

Index